Essential Medicines *for* Gastro-Intestinal Diseases

[*Homoeopathic and Patent Ayurvedic Medicines*]

Dr. S. GHOSH

Essential Medicines *for* Gastro-Intestinal Diseases

[*Homoeopathic and Patent Ayurvedic Medicines*]

Dr. SHANKAR GHOSH

G.A.M.S., D.N., D.H.M.S., D.P.T.

Specialist in Gastro-Intestinal Diseases

To be had of :

NEW CENTRAL BOOK AGENCY (P) Ltd.

8/1 CHINTAMONI DAS LANE, CALCUTTA 700 009 (INDIA)

Essential Medicines for
Gastro-Intestinal Diseases

First Published : **1998**

Publisher : Arunabha Sen
BOOKS AND ALLIED (P) Ltd.
8/1 Chintamoni Das Lane, Calcutta 700 009

Typesetter & Printer : NEW CENTRAL BOOK AGENCY (P) Ltd.
8/1 Chintamoni Das Lane, Calcutta 700 009

Cover Printer : GRAPHITECH INDIA LIMITED
Block BP, Sector V, Salt Lake, Calcutta 700 091

ISBN 81-87134-16-X

Price : Rs.**55.00** (Rupees Fifty-five) only

Preface

This BOOK is the fruit of my several years of experience, and it is prepared keeping in view the practicing knowledge requirements of the Medical Students, General Practitioners and the Self-practitioners.

Since this book, unlike other available books, deals mostly with Acute and Critical diseases of the digestive system, I am confident that those who will use this book would find new account of medicine, new system of treatment, and, above all, a source of hope and strength in their hands.

I wish the Homeopathic and Ayurvedic practitioners a success in their profession.

Christmas Day
25 December, 1997

Dr S Ghosh

Contents

Section I

Section II

Section I

ABDOMINAL PAIN

Abdominal pain may be denoted as stomach pain—is very common to all. Simple abdominal pain is not a frightening one but some abdominal pains—neglected as a simple pain of stomach problem or indigestion and subdued by a pain-killing medicine—may be a signal of a very serious abdominal disease.

Simple or serious, acute or chronic, stomach pain should never be neglected. The intensity of the pain may be so severe that the patient can die. Stomach pains are really horrible. So, whatever be the pain, a thorough investigation by the doctor is essential.

The causes of the Abdominal pain are:

1. A lump or tumour in stomach, esophagus etc.
2. Carcinoma in the stomach.
3. Ulcer in the stomach.
4. External or internal stomach injury.
5. Liver cirrhosis and damage, kidney problem.
6. Gallbladder obstruction/gallstone.
7. Gastritis, infection and poison.
8. Peritonitis and pyloric obstruction.
9. Stenosis of alimentary canal.
10. Hernia, appendicitis etc.

True abdominal pain involving the viscera or any particular organ affected would be understood by the nature of the pain. The pain would radiate from the affected organ and the pain would not shift position. It may be recurrent, mild or severe, but the place of pain would be the same. But indirect abdominal pain may be position-changing, may not be felt on palpation. Indirect pain does not aggravate much, because it is dependent on the gravity of the disease or affection of the actual organ involved. For example, a renal pain may be confused with some intestinal pain, colitis, hernia, appendicitis, gastric distension etc. Similarly, a pain of liver—whether cirrhosis of liver or not—may be confused with gallbladder pain, peptic ulcer pain etc. So, in all cases of abdominal complaints, all organs of the abdomen need to be checked by a doctor. The type of pain even referred or indirect pain helps in diagnosis of the exact disease. For example, fleeting pain from gallbladder and liver region (right hypochondrium to upper portion of right lumbar) travels to the extreme of right arm, then it is a problem of gallbladder and not any pain of hand or chest. In this manner—by understanding the type of pain—a doctor can start treatment of the actual disease.

So, the treatment of the abdominal diseases would proceed according to the nature of the disease and signs and symptoms. In general, the following abdominal cases are noticed:

1. Indigestion/Dyspepsia.
2. Dysentery/Diarrhea.
3. Cholera.
4. Flatulence/Hyperacidity.
5. Mucus, Colitis/Colic.
6. Constipation/Stricture of Rectum.
7. Ulcer/Abscess.
8. Amebic Hepatitis/Viral Hepatitis/Jaundice.
9. Liver Abscess/Cirrhosis of liver.
10. Appendicitis.
11. Gallbladder inflammation/Obstruction/Stone.

12. Ascites.

13. Enteritis/Intestinal infection/Bleeding.

14. Hematemesis.

15. Others refer to causes of abdominal diseases mentioned in this chapter.

Patients of digestive problems must take simple food. fruits. fruit juice and milk. Regular simple physical exercises in open air and keeping a cheerful temperament is essential. Tobacco. wine and excessive sexual indulgence should be avoided. Sun-bask. river-bath are helpful. Latent malaria and chronic diseases. if any, should be treated.

Flow chart be entered separate next page.

ACUTE ABDOMEN

Acute abdomen refers to several abdominal complaints which reach the extreme point of expressing themselves suddenly in the form of severe pain encompassing any area, beginning from the epigastrium to the iliac region.

This sudden beginning of the pain makes the disease an acute case and it is called *Acute abdomen.* The pain is a symptom accompanied by other symptoms, such as, persistent nausea, vomiting, headache, slight fever, vertigo and spasms in the abdomen area and specially around the affected organ or organs of the abdomen.

The most important sign of acute abdomen is persistent or immediately recurring very sharp blinding pain. This pain is not a disease. Behind the pain there lies the actual disease in its extreme stage—the fatal stage.

Some Causes of Gastro Intestinal Diseases

Protozoal Parasites

- B. Coli
- Embadomona Intestinalis
- Entamoeba Coli
- Entamoeba Histolytica
- Enteronoma H
- Giardia
- Leishmania Donovani
- Trichomonas Hominis

Helminths

- Acaris Lumbricoides
- Ancylostoma Duodenale
- Diphyllobothrium Latum
- Enterobius Vermicularis
- Fasciola Hepatica
- Gastrodiscoides Hominis
- Schistosomes
- Taenia Saginata
- Taenia Solium
- Trichinella Spiralis
- Trichuris Trichiura

Others

- Lack of Exercises
- Over Sexual Activity
- Psycological
- Thyroid and Gland Problems
- Vitamin Deficiency

Food Habits

- Alcohol
- Chemical
- Food Allergy
- Foul Air, water
- Improperly Cooked—*Flesh, Vegetables*
- Over-eating
- Smoking
- Spices
- Wrong Food

→ **Bacteria**

- Escherichia Coli
- M. Tuberculosis
- Salmonellae Paratyphi
- Salmonellae Typhi
- Staphylococci Pyogens
- Streptococci Pyogens
- Vibrio Cholerae

Acute appendicitis, peritonitis, ulcer-perforation, infected or strangulated hernia, acute cholecystitis, intestinal obstruction, rupture, diverticulitis, mucus infection, acute salpingitis, typhoid etc. may be a cause of the sudden onset of pain or acute abdomen. To understand exactly the nature of the disease behind the pain, a thorough investigation of the abdomen is necessary. The place of pain, the type of pain, the intensity of pain, for example, a persistent pain in the McBurny's point in the right iliac fossa, with a feeling of lump in that place, is suggestive of acute appendicitis.

Sometimes such pains are confused with ovarian, renal or mucus colitis etc., but the other symptoms and the place of pain, the radiation of that pain etc. give a hint to the disease the patient is suffering from. Likewise, a little bulging at the epigastrium and gas collection at the upper part of diaphragm, with pain, nausea etc., is enough to predict a case of perforation of stomach and the case is established if the patient had suffered from peptic ulcer and if examination shows no peristaltic movement of the abdomen, then it is a case of acute peritonitis. In all cases of acute abdomen, if time allows, an immediate confirmation test is necessary.

X-ray, Barium-meal X-ray, Sigmoidoscopy, Cholecystography, Blood Test etc. are done, according to the requirement. Until confirmation, immediate treatment is necessary to alleviate the severe pain. So, the general pain-killers should be administered along with drugs for assumed disease.

Treatment

1. To alleviate the severe pain, treatment for both infection and inflammation should be started.

   Cuprum Sulph 6, Belladon a 6 and **Arsenic-Iod 6** should be alternately given.

or

Ferrom Phos 12x, Kali-Sulph 12x, Arsenic-Iod 12x should be alternately given.

Even **Tinospora C 1x, Piperlongum 1x, Onosmodium 1x** and **Terebinth 12x** with water is good in checking all problems associated with acute abdomen.

2. The Ayurvedic composition of **Pepper** (*Piperlongom*). **Hing** (*Asafoetida*), **Nausadar** (*Sal Ammoniac*), **Amla** (*Emblica officinalis*), **Saunf** (*Aniseed*), **Babul Bark** (*Acacia Arabica*)—all of these or a few as available be used to prepare decoction and 5 ml of decoction taken thrice daily. This would also check gastritis and flatulence.

Patent Ayurvedic Medicines

1. **Agni Kumar Ras** (Baidyanath):

   1 to 2 tablets thrice daily with water.

or

2. **Tab Gasex** (Himalaya):

   2 tablets thrice daily for pain and inflammation, indigestion.

3. **Shoolbarjini Bati** (Baidyanath):

   1 to 2 tablets along with any of the above tablets for relieving pain and inflammation.

4. **Tab Posex Forte** (Charak):

   2 to 3 tablets, 3 to 4 hourly if required to check intestinal bleeding.

5. **Syrup A. G. Forte** (Deccan Ayurved):

   1 to 2 teaspoonful thrice daily after recovery for restorative purpose A.G. Forte is a good restorative tonic 1/2 dose of adult is recommended for children and 1/4 dose for infants, if necessary.

6. Even Tab Alsarex (Charak):

2 tablets T.D.S. is good for gastritis and gastric ulcer.

Treatment should follow for 1 (*one*) month.

ACUTE ABDOMINAL HEMORRHAGE

Hemorrhage, or bleeding from the abdomen, is manifested by coffee-coloured vomiting or vomiting of pure red blood. In both cases, the condition of the patient may become critical. Dehydration, dryness of body, thirst, pallor and collapse may be noticed as the seriousness and duration of the disease increases.

Coffee-coloured vomiting may be the cause of bleeding due to peptic ulcer, carcinoma of the stomach or intestine. Pure red blood may be vomited or passed in stool due to rupture of stomach or intestine wall following any injury, bleeding from carcinoma, rupture of fibroids, tumour etc.

To confirm from which part the bleeding is taking place. Barium-meal X-ray, liver function test, gastroscopy, sigmoidoscopy etc. may be done as required.

Bright red blood in stool may also be due to bleeding piles, hence, investigation should be proper but coal-tar (black) stool is a symptom of deep stomach or intestinal bleeding. Since bleeding is fatal to life, immediate treatment is necessary.

Treatment

1. **Ice** compression be applied on stomach.

2. **Ferrum Iod 6x** alternately with combined 15 drops of **Hamemelis Q** and **Geranium Macu Q** in 15 to 30 minutes gap.

or

3. **Mangifora indica 1x, Erigeron 1x** alternately.

4. **Vipera 30** in chronic cases.

5. Decoction prepared with the following or the direct juice are helpful—5 ml thrice daily or several times—**Lajwanti** (*Mimosa Pudica*), **Gule Abbas** (*Morabilis Jalapa*), **Satawar** (*Asparagus Race*), **Banyan** (*Ficus Bengalanis*), **Lahi** (*Lac/Cateria Lacca*).

6. Other drugs for controlling of bleeding are: **Acalypha indica, Ergot, Adrenaline, Hydrastin-mur** and **Trillium.**

Patent Ayurvedic Medicines

1. **Tab Styplon** (Himalaya):

   2 tablets with water 4 (*four*) hourly till bleeding stops.

or

2. **Cap Humeral** (Indo-German):

   2 caps with water thrice daily.

or

3. **Tab Posex Forte** (Charak):

   2 to 3 tablets thrice daily.

Note: Any two different tablets can be combined and taken depending on the direction of Physician.

ACUTE APPENDICITIS

Acute appendicitis is the inflammation of the appendix, which is an appendage or extension of the cecum. When the interior or hollow of the appendix is blocked by any outside substances such as fecal matter, purulent mucus, worms etc., then the appendix gets inflamed, swells and becomes very painful. Sometimes, in simple inflammation, the pain may subside within 48 (*forty-eight*) hours and recur time to time for several months, even years. This type may be called *chronic appendicitis*. If the inflammation does not subside within 48 (*forty-eight*) hours then the appendicitis is a serious one and infection by bacteria are generally feared.

The symptoms of severe pain in the right iliac fossa preceded by nausea and vomiting is a sign of acute appendicitis (non-obstructive). But if the pain is very severe, with violent bouts of vomiting and nausea and a contracting feeling in the cecum, it is a case of acute appendicitis (*obstructive*). This obstructive type is very dangerous as it may lead to bursting or perforation of the appendix and spreading of the pus, purulent matter outside the appendix. As a consequence peritonitis, sepsis, gangrene may begin. So, for combating this fatal disease, the following treatment is necessary.

Treatment

1. To check septic and the expected spread of infection, use **Pyrogen 30.** On nonavailability of this medicine **Echinesea 3x** or **Acid Carb 200** or **Arsenic 30** or **Mag Sulph 6x** or **Myristica Sebi 3x.**

2. To check inflammation and pain immediately **Belladona 6x** and **Iris Tenex 6x** alternately or in mixed form—both effective—or compound of **Tamarix Dioica Q** and **Gardenia Gummafera Q.**

   Treatments 1 and 2 would check the problems of acute appendicitis.

3. In place of treatment 2, the following medicines can also be used—**Achyranthes Aspera 3x, Berberis Aqui 3x.**

4. Decoction prepared by boiling the following 10 ml 3 times daily is beneficial.

   a) **Rasaut** (*Berbesis*)*
   Long pepper (*Piper Longom*)
   Harishnagar (*Night Jasmine*)
   Nausadar (*Salmiac*)
   Baoberang (*Embelia Ribes*)
   Babul (*Acacia Arabica*)*

   or

   b) **Nausadar** (*Sal Ammon*)
   Deekamali (*Gardenia Gummifera*)*
   Talwar Phali (*Cassia Occidentalis*)
   Gauma Booti (*Leucas Cephalotes*)*
   Pudina (*Mint leaves*)

Patent Ayurvedic Medicines

1. **Karamati Tablet** (Rajbaidh Sitalprasad):

   2 tablets with water to check both inflammation and pain.

2. **Shoolbarjini Bati** (Baidyanath):

   2 tablets thrice daily to check pain and inflammation.

3. **Pranda Syrup** (Baidyanath):

   1 to 2 teaspoonful thrice daily to check inflammation and temperature.

4. In combination with treatment 1:

   Special T.B. Injection (Bundelkhand):

   1 injection daily to be given in serious cases for better result.

5. **Anantamool Injection** (Sidhi):

1 injection daily to check the inflammation. It should be given if necessary.

or

6. **Sarsaparilla Syrup** (Zandu):

2 teaspoonful thrice daily or 3 (*three*) hourly, if necessary, to check inflammation.

ACUTE PANCREATITIS

Acute Pancreatitis is also a serious abdominal disease. It is the combined case of malfunctioning of the pancreas and inflammation thereof.

Malfunctioning or cessation of the proper production of the pancreatic enzymes is due to the formation of stone in the biliary tract, stricture of the tract due to inflammation, abscess etc. Inflammation is caused by the infection, acid, alcohol etc. and by the retrograde effect of malfunctioning of pancreas.

Intense pain in the epigastrium radiating to the surrounding areas, chest and back, with the sign that most pancreatic pain is aggravated after taking food and this pain is not relieved by taking antacid drugs. Besides this vomiting or nausea, slight rise in temperature, reeling of head, weight loss (in chronic case) are seen.

Stool test, blood test and X-ray are generally necessary to confirm the case.

Treatment

1. Bed rest or hospitalisation.

2. Glucose water or I V saline, if necessary.

3. For bleeding from pancreas specific treatment must simultaneously begin.

4. For diabetic patients appropriate antidiabetic medicine may be administered.

5. **Cochlera 6, Belladona 6,** or **Atropia Sulph 6x** be administered or (*Cuprum Ars* 6, *Belladona* 6, *Mag Phos* 6x) combined are effective. **Cobaltum 30** or **Vipera 200** for pain and inflammation. **Aurum Mur Nat 30, Ceanothus 1x, Taraxacum 1x, Theridon 30** for hypertrophy of the pancreas. **Carbo-Animalis 200** be given importance.

6. **Tinospora Cordifolia 1x, Aegle folia 1x** (*only in dropsy cases*), **Caesalpinia Bondu 1x** (*individually*) are effective.

7. The composition of **Gauna Booti** (*Leucas Cephalotes*), **Giloy** (*Tinospora Cordifolia*), **Pepper** (*Piper Longum*), **Hing** (*Asafoetida*), **Bathwa** (*Chenopodium*) 10 ml of decoction 3 times a day.

Patent Ayurvedic Medicines

1. **Liv-dap** (Deccan):

   2 teaspoonful thrice daily.

2. **Shoolbarjini Bati** (Baidyanath):

   1 tablet in combination with above thrice daily.

3. **Anantamool Injection** (Sidhi):

    1 injection daily in acute inflammation.

4. **Pippalimul Churna** (Zandu):

    10 to 25 grain thrice daily.

5. **Apamarg Injection** (Bundelkhand):

    1 injection daily is a supportive treatment.

ACUTE PERITONITIS

Acute peritonitis is one of the causes of acute abdomen. If untreated immediately it can cost life. Acute peritonitis is caused by organisms such as *E. coli, B. coli, B. proteus*, Strepto and Staphylococci, Gonococci and other pyogenic organisms.

Other causes are the intestinal wounds, abscess, appendicitis, carcinoma, etc., which all may cause severe inflammation of the peritoneum, serve abdominal pain, abdominal muscle rigidity, vomiting, lack of peristaltic movement, high pulse beat (slow pulse rate) in last stage and temperature, etc. are sure indication of peritonitis.

Treatment

1. Immediate hospitalisation.

2. Locating the cause and resorting to treatment.

3. Sucking out the obstructed and putrifying contents of the stomach and intestine, also administering enema to clear the bowels.

4. Liquid diet/orange juice/glucose water.

5. Saline and oxygen may be necessary.

6. In obstructive and perforated abdominal peritonitis. operation becomes essential.

7. The following medicines are required:

   Cuprum Ars 6, Belladona 6, Ferrum Phos 12x combined, or **Cuprum Ars, Terebinth, Mag Phos**—all potency are effective.

   Cuprum Ars may be substituted by **Terramycin 30,** or **Streptomycin 30,** or **Chloromycetin 30** in all cases of pain, peritonitis, or infection.

   To overcome any obstruction in bowel use plumbum met 6, alternately with chinni sulph 6 or ignatia 30, senecio 6, bryonia 30 and kali phos 30 to correct stomach hardness.

   To decoction prepared from **Gauma Booti** (*Leucas Cepalotes*), **Hing** (*Asafoetida*), **Giloy** (*Tinospora Cordifolia*), **Amla** (*Emblica officinalis*), **Ajawan** (*Ptychotis Ajowan*) and also extracts of **Babul Bark** (*Acacia Arabica*). **Hing** (*Asafoetida*) and **Ajawan** (*Ptychotis Ajowan*) relieves pain and spasm of stomach and intestine.

Patent Ayurvedic Medicines

1. **Shoolkesari Capsule** (Mishra):

   2 capsules thrice daily.

or

2. **Shoolkesari Injection** (Mishra):

   1 to 2 ml twice daily.

3. **Pirahar Tablet** (Rajbaid Sitalprasad):

   2 tablets 4 (*four*) hourly for some days.

4. **Anantamool Injection** (Bundelkhand):

   1 ml twice daily along with any above treatment for better result.

5. **Blood Purifier Syrup** (Zandu):

   It is useful for all sorts of inflammation, infections.

6. **Jwar Sanghar Capsule** (Mishra):

   1 tablet thrice daily for checking rising temperature and intestinal inflammation.

7. **Prabalpisti Injection** (Mishra):

   1 or 2 ml intramuscular if the patient goes into syncope, or loses consciousness.

General Tips

1. **To induce vomiting:**

   Ipecac 1x 20 drops or more according to the seriousness of the case.

   or

   Apomorphia 6x or **3x** 10 drops with water, if necessary may be repeated.

   or

   Powdered mustard seed and half teaspoon of salt with a glass of water.

2. **To delay absorption of Poison and Acid:**

   Give charcoal powder (30 gm) with water or slaked lime water.

   White of egg (approximately 10 to 11 eggs) be fed, preferably with flour added in water.

2

or

Magnesium Sulphate having the property to counter poison or toxin should also be fed.

3. To induce urination:

If urine has stopped—A compound of **Ammonium Mur 6x,** or **Ammonum Chloride, Soda bicarb** and **Potassium Chloride** (*Kalimur* 3x) be given in 20 to 30 minuites gap.

The combined Ayurvedic drugs—**Purnanava** (*Boerhavea Diffusa*) and **Biranjashif** (*Achilea Milefolium*) are diuretic, even **Gokhru** (*Tribulus terrestris*).

AMEBIASIS

Amebiasis or mucus infection, as may be called, is caused by the organism Entameba Histolytica.

Gastro-entero problems of colitis, cramps, mucus and bloody stool, flatulence, dyspepsia and, lastly, in chronic cases, can lead to formation of abscess and ulcers in liver and intestine.

Treatment

Cuprum Acete 6 or **Emetine 6x** or 6 alternately with **Atista-indica 1x**—also refer to chapter on dysentery for more symptoms and treatment. In general, **Kuruchi 1x, Bismuth 6x, Iodoformum 6** alternately are most effective.

ASCITES

It is also known as *Abdominal dropsy.* Ascites or abdominal dropsy is the free fluid collection in the peritoneal cavity.

It may manifest as a swelling of the abdomen and shrinking of the muscles of the body or it may be swelling of the abdomen as well as the body. But in any type there is the fluid in the peritoneal cavity. The gurgling sound of the fluid can be heard.

The cause of this ascites disease are:

1. Cirrhosis of liver.
2. Nephritis (*indirectly*).
3. Congestive heart failure.
4. Obstruction of the portal veins.
5. Other problems of the peritoneum including infection, adjoining tumour, carcinoma, thrombosis etc.

Treatment

1. Bed rest.
2. For mild ascites treatment may cure it.
3. For massive ascites, surgical drainage of the fluid is necessary—then followed by other treatments.
4. **Apocynum can 3x, Kati Nitrium 6, Mercurius sol 30** alternately in preliminary cases.
5. **Kali Carb 12x, Acid flurica 30, Apis Mel 6** alternately also effective in hard liver. **Myristica Sebi 3x** and **Coleus Aroma 1x-Apocynum 1x** combined taken thrice with any of the above is effective in ascites.

Patent Ayurvedic Medicines

1. **Jalodarari Ras** (Sidhi):

   1 tablet once or twice daily to check ascites.

or

2. **Punarnavadi Guggulu** (Sidhi):

   2 to 3 tablets once daily. It is good in dropsy and it is a diuretic.

or

3. **Jalodarari Injection** (Mishra):

   1 or 2 injections daily or alternative day.

4. **Liv 52** (Himalaya):

   2 tablets twice daily be taken along with any of the above treatment.

5. **Lauh Basma** (Dabur) and **Ramban Ras** (Baidyanath):

   Jointly is good for ascites and dropsical cases.

Note: Purnanara (*Buerhaavia Diffusa*) **1x** and **Gokhru** (*Tribulus Terrestis*) **1x** helps to expel collected fluid and reduce all sorts of edema.

The other wonderful remedies for ascites following cirrhosis of liver are Boerhaavia diffusa. Caesalpinia bonducella Q. Hydrocotyle asiatica Q. Hygrophilia spinosa Q. All these are also recommened for any type of liver spleen complaints.

Decoction prepared from the following are efficient in healing ascites. 10 ml 4 times daily.

Purnarva (*Trianthem monogyme*)*.

Guruch (*Tinospora Cordi*)*.

Daruhaldi (*Berberis Sp.*).

Kutki (*Picrorhiza Kurrora*).

Parvas Patra (*Trichosanthes Dioica*).

Neem Bask (*Azadirachta Indica*)*.

Debdaru (*Cedrus Deodara*).

Standard drugs are **Jalodarari Rasa, Ichchovedi Rasa.**

CHOLERA

Cholera is a fatal disease caused by the organism called *Vibrio-cholerae,* disrupting the entire gastro-intestinal functions. The main symptoms are rice-water stool, so loss of body fluid, abdominal cramps, initially fast pulse, later slowing of pulse and collapse, then ice-cold body and even death.

Treatment

On the basis of the symptoms such as rice-water stool the treatment should begun. Stool test is also necessary. **Cuprum Ars 6x** or 6 alternately with **Jatropha 6x** is best or **Cuprum Ars** combined with **Chinrinum Sulph 6** be given alternately with **Mercurius Dulchis 6. Acid-Hydro 6** for increasing the body heat and pulse in stage of collapse. Also refer to chapter on diarrhea for other symptoms.

CIRRHOSIS OF LIVER

It is a stage of hypertrophy and degeneration of liver cells. If liver cells come in contact with toxic substances even hepatitis B infection, or due to fatty degeneration of liver the hepato-cellular function of the liver is impaired and degeneration or cirrhosis of liver is said to have taken place.

The symptoms of jaundice such as the yellow discoloration of skin may not be there but nausea, indigestion, disgust for food. Sexual disturbances, anorexia and loss of weight are enough to suggest some serious ailment of liver.

Liver pain, heaviness feeling in liver region, oedema in the lower body parts specially around ankles and, in extreme cases, Ascites are absolute confirmation that the liver ailment is nothing but cirrhosis of liver.

Blood test for serum bilirubin, alkaline phosphatase, hemoglobin, albumin-globulin etc. even liver biopsy is helpful test for confirmation of the degree of cirrhosis including liver carcinoma.

Treatment

1. Bed rest and immediate hospitalisation preferred.
2. In ascites drainage of the fluid is first necessary. In preliminary case of ascites.
3. In blood vomiting use juice of **Lajwanti** (*Mimosa Pudika*) or **Goksura** (*Tribulus Rerrestris*) **powder, Ipepac 6x, Geranium Mac 1x, Erigeron 1x** (*together*) be given.
4. Diuretics may be required. Refer chapter of Jaundice and Ascites.
5. Anti-anemic medicines as a **Ferrum-Mur 6, Alfalfa Q, Zincum Met 30** be given.
6. Glucose/Fruit juice diet is necessary.
7. Proper medicines to control intestinal infection such as Vaccinum **Myrtillus 6x, Baptisa 3x, Chloromycetin 30, Arsenic Sulph Rub 30**—any of these may be used thrice a day.

8. The juice or decoction of **Bhringaraha** (*Eclipta Alba*), **Kutki** (*Picrorhizakurrora*), **Arjuna** (*Terminalia Arjuna*)*, **Purnarva** (*Boerhaavia*-Diffusa*) 10 ml taken 3 times daily and take salt-free diet.

Patent Ayurvedic Medicines

1. **Gastrodap** (Deccan):

   1 to 2 tablets thrice for indigestion, nausea, flatulence, loss of appetite.

2. **Liv-dap** (Deccan):

   2 to 3 teaspoonful thrice for sluggish liver, hepatitis, liver inflammation etc.

or

3. **Livomyn Drops** (Charak):

   2 teaspoonful thrice daily for Hepatitis, cirrhosis of liver, sluggish liver.

or

4. **Arogyavardhini Tablets** (Baidyanath):

   1 to 2 tablets with water thrice for all liver disorder.

5. **Jalodari Ras Tablets** (Sidhi):

   1 tablet once daily in case of ascite and related symptoms.

Note: In case of Ascites besides conventional medicines, Diuretic such as Punarnavarishta of any Ayurvedic company should be used.

CONSTIPATION AND FLATULENCE

It is a common case with most people leading a sedentary life. Due to physical weakness, anemia and digestive disorder. The evacuation of the waste matter from the bowels does not take place. Sometimes lack of contractility of the bowels causes constipation, which, in turn, leads to several health problems.

When the collected waste matter putrefies, gas or flatulence is resulted causing pain and distress.

Treatment

The decoction prepared by rose petals and sennă leaves and aniseed is the best for relieving of constipation and, consequently, flatulence. The power of **Hing** (*Asafoetida*), **Black Salt, Ambla** (*Emblica officinalis*) is very effective for checking gas or wind accumulation in stomach. Standard medicines are **Avipittakar Churna, Swadishta Virechan.** In homeopathy, constipation is relieved by **Hydrastis 1x** (twice daily), **Nux-vom 30** alternately with **Bryonia 200** (twice daily), **Lae-Defl 30** in the evening or **Rhammus Cali 1x** or **Cascara Sag 1x**. 10–15 drops twice daily with lukewarm water. **Senna 1x** 15–20 drops with lukewarm water at bed time in evening. For flatulence refer to chapter on Dyspepsia.

Patent Ayurvedic Medicines

1. Herbolax Tablet (Himalaya):

2 to 3 tablets with lukewarm water at night, bed time.

2. Regulax Tablet (Charak):

2 tablets with water or milk at night, bed time.

3. Laxodap Tablet (Deccan):

2 tablets at night, bed time, with warm milk or water.

4. Kostbadhati Bati (Rajbaid Sitalprasad):

2 tablets at night, bed time, with warm water or milk.

5. Kabz-Har (Dabur):

2 teaspoonful with warm water or milk at night, bed time.

Any of the above can be selected.

DIARRHEA

Diarrhea, as the name suggests, is the sudden inflammation of stomach and the intestines causing frequent evacuation of the contents of the stomach and the intestine. This act of evacuation is sparked-off by the body's defence mechanism to eliminate the toxin that has entered the alimentary system, the stomach and intestine which may eventually enter the blood.

Diarrhea is caused by:

1. Food poison.

2. Excess acid formation in stomach.

3. Viral infection.

4. Bacterial infections, e.g., *Escheria coli, B. coli*, etc. and even other bacteria migrating from urinary tracts to intestines.

5. Protozoal, e.g., worms, giardia etc.

6. Allergy, Reaction to some drugs etc.

The symptoms are loose watery stool, with or without undigested food particles, with or without cramping pain and vomiting. Diarrhea is to be feared because it leads to loss of body fluids and essential salts from the body. The patient may collapse, even death can occur.

Treatment

1. After checking for the dryness of the body surface, in other words, if the skin and lips look dry, parched, severe loss of fluid or dehydration has taken place and patient's condition may prove fatal, then immediate administration of oral Rehydration salts are to be made. And for the unconscious patients intravenous saline has to be administered.

2. Blood pressure and pulse rate should be checked time to time.

3. The medicines are:

   Kuruchi Q and **Atista Indica 6x** (mixed up) 5 drops 4 times is effective or **Asarum Eup 3x, Kurchi 3x,** or **Podophyllum 3x** (mixed up) or **Merc-Dulchis 6** alternately with **Cuprum Ars 6.**

4. **Cuphea 1x, Liatris Spiceta 3x, Cyperus Rotindus 1x, Hydrocotyl Asiatica 1x, Luffa Amara 1x** are also effective individually or mixed up.

5. **Camphor 6, Carbo-veg 6, Arsenic 6** and **China 6** needed in case of body becoming cold.

In the treatment of diarrhea the following composition is effective: The decoction of Kuruchi (*Holarrhena Antidysenterica*), Babul (*Acacia Arabica*), Hing (*Asafoetida*) with or without Dhayfool (*Woodfordia Floribonda*) be taken 4 times a day. The composition of Dhania (*Corriandum*), Pepper (*Piper Longum*). Jaifal (*Croton Tigilum*) small amount, Kuruchi (*Hola-Andidysentrica*) is very good.

Patent Ayurvedic Medicines

1. **Deepan Tablet** (Charak):

   2 tablets thrice daily till cured.

2. **Diadyn Syrup** (Charak):

   2 teaspoonful thrice daily till cured.

3. **Posex Forte Tab** (Charak):

   2 tablets thrice daily to check bleeding, if any, and, if necessary, in acute cases.

4. **Shoolbarjini Bati** (Baidyanath):

   1 to 2 tablets 4 (*four*) hourly to check cramps and pain.

5. **Prandata Tablet** (Amritdhara):

   Very effective in serious conditions.

6. **Cholera Injection** (Bundelkhand):

   2 ml intramuscular 4 (*four*) hourly in case of cholera or cholera-like diarrhea.

7. **Bisuchikantak Injection** (Mishra):

   2 ml 1m (on waiste) 3 to 4 (*four*) hourly till result obtained.

DYSENTERY (ORDINARY AND BACILLARY)

Ordinary dysentery is generally referred as amebic dysentery, which leads to great cramping pain and frequent purging. The stool is loaded with mucus, undigested food substances, but no blood. It is because of the infection of the large instestine, sometimes spreading to the small intestine.

But it is not to be feared, except when it is bacillary or blood dysentery, which has the symptoms of dysentery, but these would be blood in the stool. Stool test confirms the presence of *shigella group of bacteria.* This disease is serious as, along with the body fluid, blood is also drained out making the patient too weak and condition fatal.

Treatment

Chloromycetin 30, alternately with the mixture of **Atista indica 1x, Geranium Mac, Emetine 6x** or mixture of **Acacia Arabica 1x, Hydrocotyl Asiatic 1x,** and **Merc Dulchis 6** incurrently. **Euphorbia 3x, Hydras Mur 6x** (one one) are also effective.

To cure bacillary and blood dysentry, nateuropaths can use the compound prepared with **Kutz** (*Holarrhena-Antidy Sentrica*), **Babul** (*Acacia Arabica*), **Mukatabarshi** (*Acalypha Indica*), **Ash-sheora** (*Atista Radix*) or **Telakucha-Bimba** (*Cephalandra Indica*). About a cup of the extract or decoction 3 times a day. The standard drugs are **Kutajaghana Vati** or **Piyushavalli Rasa.**

Patent Ayurvedic Medicines

1. **Diarex Tablet** (Himalaya):

   1 tablet thrice daily, in extreme cases 2 tablets thrice daily. Children 1/2 of adult dose.

2. **Dysentrina Tablet** (Mehta):

   2 tablets 4 (*four*) hourly till cured.

3. **Deepan Tablet** (Charak):

   2 tablets thrice daily.

4. **Diadyn Syrup** (Charak):

   2 teaspoonful 3 to 4 times daily, 1/2 dose for children and 1/4 dose for infants.

5. **Kutja Syrup** (Deccan):

   2 teaspoonful thrice daily.

6. **To overcome weakness A.G. Forte Syrup** (Deccan):

   Should be administered for some days.

DYSPEPSIA

Dyspepsia is another word of indigestion. It is very common among people. The symptoms are bloating of stomach after food, sour eructation, nausea, even vomiting, pain after food, flatulence, irregular stool evacuation, with or without mucus stool test show undigested food particles. Sluggishness of liver activity is always present in dyspepsia.

Treatment

Timely and unspiced food should be taken with the compositon of **Nux-vom 1x, Carbo-veg 1x, Pepsinum 1x** after food or just **Nux-vom 1x** alternately with **Caujuputum 3x,** or **Gaultheria 3x,** or **Iris-vers 1x** (*for acid formation*). Also **Amloki Q** and **Alfalfa Q** are good.

Patent Ayurvedic Medicines

1. **Alsarex Tablet** (Charak):

   It is an antacid, prevents esophageal reflux, epigastric pain, dyspepsia. 2 tablets thrice daily.

2. **Gastrodap Tablet** (Deccan Ayurvedic):

   1 to 2 tablets twice daily to check indigestion, nausea, acidity, flatulence and loss of appetite.

3. **Agnitundi Bati** (Dabur):

   2 tablets thrice daily to check above-mentioned complaints.

4. **Livomyn Drops** (Charak):

   1 to 2 teaspoonful thrice daily to correct liver sluggishness even cirrhosis of liver, if any. 1/2 dose for children and 1/4 dose for infants.

5. **Raktoy Syrup** (Deccan):

   1 to 2 teaspoonful to overcome anemia.

6. **Crominill Syrup** (Charak):

   2 to 3 teaspoonful thrice daily for 3 (*three*) days to expel worms, 1/2 dose for children.

DYSPHAGIA

This is also a serious disease. It constitutes esophageal pain, inflammation and difficulty in swallowing food and drinks. It is a matter of serious concern, as no food and drinks pass through the esophagus without causing distressing pain and spasm, which is due to the constriction or narrowing or stricture or stenosis as may be called of the esophagus. This narrowing may begin from the throat and lead downward into the alimentary canal.

The common cause of this problem may be inflammation and swelling of the food passage due to tonsilitis diphtheria, pharangitis etc. or due to external material stuck up in the throat. Tumour, abscess, bronchial infections, hydrophobia, cancer of the affected area etc. are also important causes. Barium X-ray of esophagus is necessary.

Treatment

1. Choked and constricted feeling in the esophagus—**Abies Can 6x, Anacardium 6, Canabis Sativa 6,** two of these be used alternately.

or

2. Feeling of heaviness, spasm, with constriction, then Cuprum **Acetic 6, Lauroserus 6, Hyasyamus 30, Kali Bich 200, Gelsemium 200,** two of these alternately be used.
3. Contraction with pain—Any one medicine of the above and **Ammon Mur 200**, or **Agaricus 200.**
4. Constriction with hardening of the esophageal muscles—**Plumbum-Iod 200, Polygonum Ar 6x, Graphitis 200, Senecio 30**, any two alternately used.
5. For constriction due to infections, use **Merc-Bin-Iod 30,** (*Phytolecca Q Echinesia Q*) for gurgle and 6x of both internally, **Pyrogen 200** and **Arsenic-Iod 30** should be first used in 1 (*one*) hour gap.
6. For presence of fleshy lumpin the food passage use Cal-flue 1m, B. Carb 1m or Cal-Iod 1m.
7. Argent Met 200, Cocculus 30, Belladona 200, Zinc Phos 30 in chronic cases be tried.
8. In confirmed case the treatment should be with **Condurango 3x, Phytolacca 3x and Carcinosin 30.**

Patent Ayurvedic Medicines

1. **Pirahar Tablet** (Rajbaid Sitalprasad):

   2 tablets thrice daily for some days.

2. **Pinex Tablet** (Charak):

   2 tablets thrice for some days alone or in combination of 1 tablet of Pirahar.

3. **Bathbidar Injection** (Mishra):

   1 injection daily to overcome muscular rigidity and tightness.

4. **Aparijita Injection** (Bundelkhand):

   1 ml twice or on alternative day to reduce throat inflammation.

5. **Dicronil Liquid** (Charak):

   2 teaspoonful to check esophageal and bronchial spasm, inflammation.

FISTULA IN ANO

A fistula or canal formed between the rectum and the anus due to the formation of abscess. The abscess is formed around the anus and engulfs the region of the rectum, making an extra-link or canal between the rectum and the anus.

The disease is marked by muco-purulent discharges or just discharges of pus and blood, pain and swelling of that region. If the fistula is not immediately treated it can lead to pyaesia and even paralysis of rectum.

Treatment

1. **Arsenic-Iod 200, Acid Mur 200** and **Silecia 6x** alternately. **Arsenic-Iod** and **Acid Mur 2** times and **Silecia 4** times a day or **Myristica Sebi 3x.**

or

2. **Polygonun 1x, Graphitis 30, Euphorbium off 6, Camocladia 6** are effective.

3. Decoction prepared by **Haldi** (*Turmeric*), **Chita** (*Plumbago Zeylanica*), **Khulekara** (*Hygrophila Spinosa*), **Haritki** (*Termenila Chebu*), **Apamarga** (*Achyranthes Aspera*) 10 ml thrice daily. The same preparation be applied externally if possible. Standard drugs such as **Brangajankush Rasa** or **Saptabisantik googul** be taken thrice daily.

4. Externally **Geranium Mac 1x** mixed with **Cistus can 1x** or **Myristica Sebi 2x** be applied. Medicines can be applied deeply by *enema* process.

Patent Ayurvedic Medicines

1. **Kapina Tablet** (Himalaya):

   2 tablets thrice daily for about 1 (*one*) month.

2. **Karamati Tablet** (Rajbaid Sitalprasad):

   2 tablets thrice or 1 tablet twice along with Kapina tablet.

3. **Healer Ointment** (Baidyanath):

   For local application.

4. **Karamati Ointment** (Rajbaid Sitalprasad):

   For local application. .

5. **Anantamool Injection** (Sidhi):

   1 injection alternative days, if required, for better result.

6. **Poxes Forte Tablet** (Charak):

   To check related bleeding 2 tablets thrice daily.

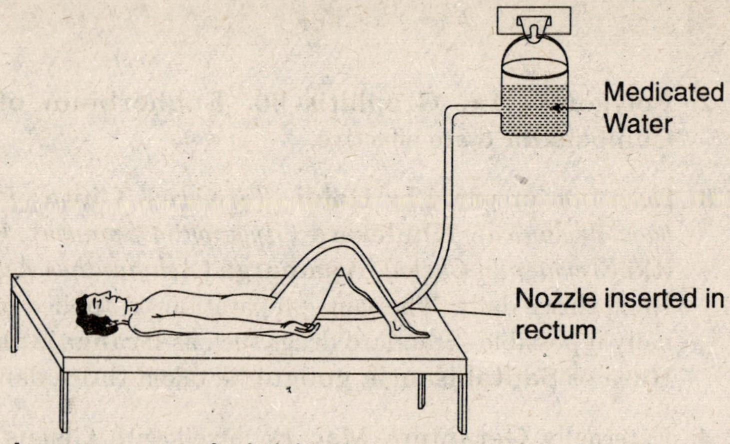

Improper way of administering enema.

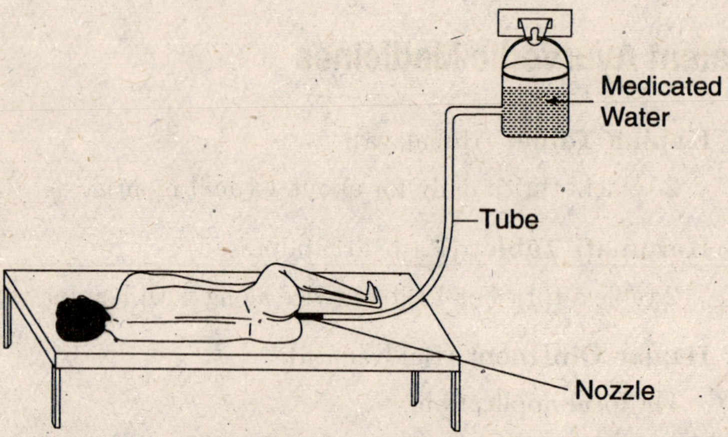

Correct way of administering enema.

Note: Enema should be taken early morning in empty stomach. Lukeworm water added with lime juice for relieving constipation. Any other medicine can be mixed with lukewarm water and taken after cleaning the bowel with plain enema for curing of colitis, peritonitis T.B., carcinoma of large intestine and also to cure piles, etc.

GALLBLADDER INFLAMMATION AND STONES

Gallbladder inflammation and gallbladder stone is a common abdominal disease. If there is no stone but acute inflammation then stabbing pain is felt in the gallbladder region encompassing the right hypochondrium epigastrium and the lower portion of the right side chest. The pain may travel across the chest to the right arm and neck. If this type of pain continues to radiate up to the arm, scapula and neck, then there is a certainty of stone formation in the gallbladder. Nausea and vomiting is common. Otherwise, pain may be due to the obstruction of the biliary tract, infection, pyogenic abscess, ulcers, cancer, cyst, etc.

Gallbladder problems become serious in the following circumstances:

1. Obstruction of the biliary tract/cystic duct.

2. Cyst and tumour formation.

3. Passage of stone via the tract causing severe pain with or without bleeding.

4. Formation of abscess or fistula or cancer.

5. Cessation of the function due to the above causes.

To understand the nature of the problem, cholecystography and blood test should be done.

If medicine does not relieve the disease early and if the cholecystography shows the size of the stones relatively large in size then operation has to be done.

If Homeopathic medicines are regularly used, gallbladder stone formation would stop and if the size of the stones are small, then such stones too would be expelled out of the bladder.

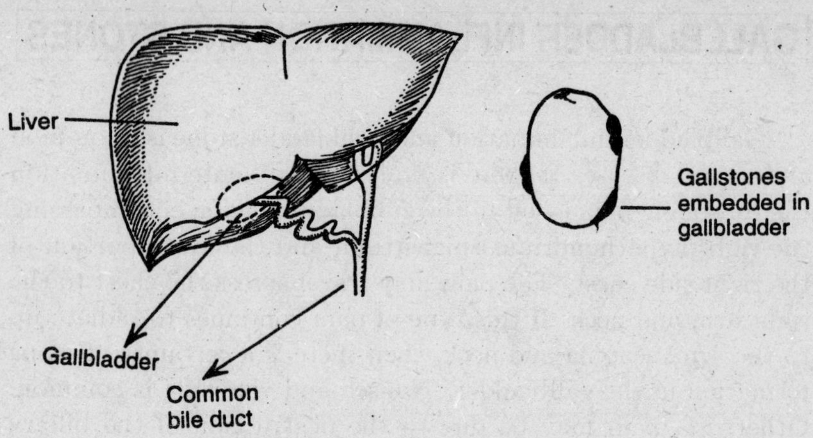

Gallbladder with stone formation.

Treatment

1. In acute pain of gallbladder with inflammation or with stones, use alternately the following medicines **Euphorbia 6, Natrum Nitri 30** and **Cobaltum 30** or **Mag-Sulph 6.**

2. To loosen the congestion and expel the stones **Taraxacum 3x,** preceded by **Atropia Sulph 12x** and **Chelidonium 3x. Lithium Carb 6** to be tried last or **Berberis Vul 1x.**

3. To induce secretion after the main treatment **Nux-Moschus 200, Podophyllum 30** or **Berberis Vul 6x,** any 2 alternately.

4. **China Q, Cardus Mari Q, Chelidonium Q** combined alternately with **Aurum Mur Nat 30** has expelled and prevented recurrence of stone.

5. **Decoction of Muli*** (*Raphanus Sativa*), **Bathwa** (*Chenopodium*), **Karanjwa*** (*Fever Nut*), **Pashan Ved*** (*Saxifraga L*), **Jawakhar** (*Pearl ash*) 10 ml thrice daily.

6. Boiled lukewarm methi water is very good.

Patent Ayurvedic Medicines

1. **Shoolbarjini Bati** (Baidyanath):

   1 to 2 tablets 3 (*three*) hourly to check pain.

2. **Tamara Bhasma** (Baidyanath):

   65 mg twice daily to check gallstone problems and liver disorder.

3. **Avipathikar Churna** (Dabur):

   1 teaspoonful when required to check acidity, gastritis and constipation.

4. **Liv Dap Syrup** (Deccan Ayurvedic):

   2 teaspoonful thrice daily in case of sluggish liver splenomegaly, infective hepatitis.

5. **Calicurry Tablet** (Charak):

   2 tablets with water thrice daily for all types of stone.

6. **Pashanbed Injection** (Bundelkhand):

   1 injection 1m daily for some days, alternately with any tablet for 1 (*one*) month.

7. **Tab Cystone** (Himalaya):

   2 tablets with lukewarm water thrice daily to expel all types of stone.

8. **Ashmari Tablet** (Dhanwantari):

   2 tablets with water thrice daily to expel stones.

Any one of above 5 to 8 be selected and used and other medicines be applied according to symptoms.

HERNIA (complicated)

Hernia is a protrusin of an organ through an opening in the abdominal wall. The different types of hernia are:

1. Diaphragmatic hernia.
2. Hiatus hernia.
3. Inguinal hernia.
4. Strangulated hernia.
5. Umbilical hernia.
6. Ventral hernia.
7. Epigastric hernia etc.

In any type of hernia complication may arise and if the complications cannot be relieved by general medicine, then operation has to be resorted to. The complications arise when

1. Hernia leads to any obstruction of the function of an organ or a system.
2. When hernia becomes irreducibility that the hernia cannot be withdrawn to its normal position from the hernial sac.
3. When the protruted hernia strangles any organ or blood vessel and impairs the function of that organ and the organs depended on a particular blood vessel.
4. Fluid in the hernial sac.
5. Infection and ulcer or gangrene of the hernial sac etc.

Treatment

1. **Aconite 6** and **Hyosyamus 30** in case of incarcerated hernia. **Tabacum 6,** alternately with **Plumbum-Iod 30** in strangulated hernia. **Lycopodium 200, Cocculus 6, Aloes 30, Ferrum Phos 12x, Aesculus 6** are good. Any 2 alternately be used.

2. Decoction prepared with the following are helpful **Arund** (*Ricinus Communis*), **Giloy** (*Tinospora Cordifolia*)*, **Gokhru** (*Tribulus terrestris*)*, **Durba** (*Cynodon Dact*) 10 ml thrice daily.

Patent Ayurvedic Medicines

1. **Nityananda Ras** (Baidyanath):

   1 to 2 tablets with warm water for hernia and dilation of stomach.

HICCOUGH (NON-STOP)

Hiccough is a very painful incidence of abdominal and other neurological disorder. Hiccough is not a disease but a reflection of acute abdominal inflammation or any other neurological disorder associated with some gastro-entero problems and spasm of the respiratory tract.

Hiccough is common incidence of gastric irritation, but when the Hiccough does not stop for hours, even days, then the patients' conditions becomes serious, even death can result.

In general, the cause of hiccough is due to the following:

1. Heart burn or acidity, indigestion that leads to forcible expansion of the stomach and esophageal muscles.
2. Other causes leading to hiccough are allergy, high fever or hot body, cancer of stomach, cerebral disorder and other abominal and general infection.

Treatment

1. Hiccough caused as a reaction to long-term wrong medicines —**Cuprum Sulph 30.**
2. Hiccough caused due to great heat and inflammation of abdomen with or without gas or constipation. **Chinninum Sulph 200** alternately with **Pulsetilla 30.**
3. Non-stop Hiccough for days—**Chinnium Ars 200, Cicuta 6, Kali Brom 6.**
4. Non-stop Hiccough making the patient blue/unconscious **Kali-hydro 200, Acid hydro 200, Nux-moschus 30, Ginseng 1x, Ignatia 30** (apply any medicine and watch result in 30 minutes).

Patent Ayurvedic Medicines

1. **Gasex Tablet** (Himalaya):

   2 tablets 3 (*three*) hourly with lukewarm water.

2. **Zyme Tablet** (Zandu):

   2 tablets 4 (*four*) hourly with lukewarm water.

3. **Aparajita Injection** (Bundelkhand):

   1 injection daily along with any above treatment for serious cases.

4. Damona Injection (Sidhi):

1 injection daily along with any above treatment for serious cases.

5. Agni Sandipan Bati (Rajbaid Sitalprasad):

2 tablets thrice daily half an hour after food.

6. Mayur Chandrika Bati (Baidyanath):

1 tablet twice daily.

Other remedies for Hiccough are:

1. The burnt ash of peacock feather taken with aniseed.

2. Decoction of the following ingredients are useful:

Pepper (*Piper longum*).

Hing (*Asafoetida*).

Kutki (*Picrorhiza Kurrao*).

Ambla (*Embelia Ribes*).

Kakrasingi (*Rhus-Succedena*).

Pudina (*Metha Sp.*)

(10 ml 2 to 3 times a day.)

JAUNDICE

Jaundice is the disease associated with many other diseases such as liver dysfunction, renal failure or other problems of circulatory systems. Jaundice is identified by the yellowish colour of the urine, eyes and skin, but confirmed by the presence of bilirubin in blood test.

The presence of bilirubin in the blood is common in all types of jaundice, but in infective hepatic jaundice—along with the presence of bilirubin—there happens to be acute inflammation of liver and also damage of liver cells. Viral infection of liver is the general cause.

The viruses Hepatitis A, Hepatitis B and non-hepatitis viruses. Of these, the Hepatitis B is more dangerous as the infection infects the blood and can cause death if not immediately treated.

The symptoms of pricking pain in the liver region, vomiting, nausea, indigestion, vertigo and mild fever etc. may give an indication that the jaundice is an infective jaundice. In viral hepatic jaundice fever is the main indication, but other complications such as enlargement of liver, oedema of liver, necrosis of liver cells etc. may arise. In biliary tract obstruction—both bilirubin and bile salts circulate in blood.

If jaundice is neglected for long or suppressed by temporary cure then the untreated jaundice may lead to liver cancer in some cases. Blood test for serum bilirubin, bile salts, serum transaminases, alkaline phosphatase and Hepatitis B virus may be required.

Treatment

1. Complete bed-rest and glucose water preferred.
2. Fruit juice or light meal as diet for a long period of time even after recovery.
3. Blood test for bilirubin and others be done on a weekly basis.
4. Immunisation with **HNIG** (*Human Normal Immunoglobulin*) for Hepatitis A virus and 'HB Vax' for Hepatitis B virus jaundice.
5. To cure obstruction in bile tract **Oxalic acid 200** time to time with **Berberis Vul 1x, Chelidonium 1x, China**

3x, **Kaliphos 12x** or **Urtica Ureus 30** alternately with Podophyllum 6. Ammon Mur 30 may be tried.

6. To induce bile flow and proper liver functioning **Podophyllum 3x** in muddy coloured stool and **Chelidonium** and **Merc-Sol. 30** alternately in white coloured stool, even **Aurum Mur Nat 30** is good. **Cardus M Q, Chionanthus Q China Q** (*Mixed up*) be taken to activate liver.

7. In damaged liver **Ferrum Phos 6, Eupatorium Purf 6x, Taraxacum 3x** is good. **Tinospora Cordifolia Q** corrects liver enlargement and problems.

8. Fatty degeneration of liver would be corrected by **Cal-Ars 30, Merc-Iod 30** alternately.

9. For sluggishness due to Necrotic tendency of liver cells, use **Theridon 30,** alternately with **Agraphis Nutans 3x.**

10. Suitable diuretics namely, the combination of **Thankuni** (*Hydrocotyle Asiatica*), **Pasanbedi** (*Saxifragia Ligulata*), **Muli** (*Raphanus Sat*) or **Peepal twig** (*Ficus Religosa*) steeped in water over night be drank.

11. If ascites is seen, then it should be first cured by drainage in case of excessively big size of Ascites. In the preliminary case of ascites—refer chapter on Ascites.

12. Suitable purgatives for bowel clearance be used. In homeopathy **Natrum Sulph 6** and **Bryonia 30** alternately or **Ignatia 30** and **Senna 1x** alternately. **Senna 1x** (10 to 15 drops) with water at bed time or **Terminalia Chebula 1x** (15 to 20) drops with lukewarm water early morning, or **Rhamnus Cali 3x** 10 to 15 drops twice daily or**cascara Sag 1x** 10 to 20 drops with lukewarm water before going to bed, also **Cascarilla 3x.** Do not take too much of purgative drugs. Effects of the purgatives depends upon person to person, so dosages may increase or decrease according to patients' choice.

Decoction or even juice of the following ingredients are useful in jaundice 10 ml thrice daily.

Purnarva (*Boerhaavia Diffusa*).

Thankuni (*Hydrocotyle Asiatica*).

Kule-khara (*Hygrophila Sphinosa*).

Kalmeg (*Andrographis Paniculata*)*.

Titpolla (*Luffa Amara*).

Arjuna (*Terminalia Arjuna*)*.

Haritki (*Terminalia Chebulla*)*.

Patent Ayurvedic Medicines

1. **Arogyavardhini Tablet** (Baidyanath):

   2 tablets with water twice daily.

2. **Liv 52** (Himalaya):

   2 tablets twice daily.

or

3. **Livomyn Drops** (Charak):

   2 teaspoonful thrice daily.

4. **Gastrodap Tablets** (Deccan Ayurvedic):

   1 to 2 tablets twice daily if symptoms of indigestion, gas, acidity flatulence persists.

5. After recovery medicines such as

   Laxodap or Herbolax to check constipation and Raktoj (Deccan Ayurvedic) to overcome Anemia should be taken for some days.

6. **A.G. Forte Syrup** (Deccan):

   It is good for overcoming general weakness and lethargy.

LIVER ABSCESS

Liver abscess is a disease that is generally associated with other stomach or abdominal ailments. Pyogenic organisms from internal tuberculosis or ulcers may reach up to liver and form abscess. Similarly, those suffering from amebiasis, mucus infection, bacillary dysentery, etc. may have liver abscess if these amebias and other bacterias migrate to the liver and settle down there.

The part where such abscess is formed is filled with pus, necrosis of the liver cells starts and liver becomes painful, sluggish and enlarged. Gallbladder type of pain starts with nausea, vomiting, sinking at the pit of the stomach, indigestion and fever. If this problem continues, anemia, rigidity of abdominal muscles, fever dropsy may be noticed. Therefore, to save the patient, a quick treatment is essential.

Treatment

1. In pyaemic liver abscess, to deal with infection and pyogenic organism **Arsenic-Iod 30** and **Cistus 30** alternately or **Pyrogen 200**, even **Theridon 30** and **Vaccicinum 30** is good.

2. In amebic liver abscess use **Merc-Sulph 30**, alternately with **Emetine 6x**.

3. To deal with liver enlargement in infective cases—**Kali-Iod 30** or **Merc-bin-Iod 30, Phytolecca 3x, Chinni-Ars 6** (*combined*) and **Pyrogen 200**.

4. For liver malfunctioning leading to dropsy of body use **Kali Nitricum 6, Merc-Dulchis 30** alternately. **Apis-Mel 30** and **Apocynum 6x** is also good. Other medicines of dropsy also to be consulted. Even **Myristica Seb 3x** alternately with **Phytolecca 6x** can cure it.

5. To promote liver function, the following medicines are essential—**Natrum Phos 30, Berberis Vul 30, Taraxacum 6x** alternately or a combined dose of **Chionanthus 1x, Chelidonum 1x** and **China 1x.**

6. The composition of **Nausadar** (*Sal Ammoniac*), **Nagkesar** (*Cobras Saforon*), **Bel** (*Balsamodendron Myrrha*), **Amla** (*Embelica officinalis*), **Kutki** (*Picrorhiza Kurroa*) in syrup or powder form are effective in correcting liver enlargement and malfunctioning.

7. To correct liver abscess the decoction or powder of the following are good—**Baron*** (*Bark of Crataeva religosa*), **Arond** (*Recivus commonis*), **Bat** (*Ficus bengalensis*), **Chita*** (*Plombago Zey*), **Haritki*** (*Terminelia Chebulla*), **Goggul** (*Balsamodendron*) and **Hirankhori** (*Corchorus Fasicularis*) boiled or water steeped with the above herbs—10 ml 3 times a day.

8. The combination of **Geranium max 1x, Cistus 6x** or **Phytolecca 6x** or **Hydrastis 3x** alternately with **Anthracinum 200** is very effective.

Patent Ayurvedic Medicines

1. **Karamati Tablet** (Rajbaidh Sitalprasad):

   1 to 2 tablets with water to check abscess.

2. **Dardona Tablet** (Baidyanath):

   1 to 2 tablets if required to check pain, twice daily.

or

3. **Shoolarin Injection** (Bundelkhand):

   1 injection 1m to check pain, once daily.

or

4. **Anantamool Injection** (Sidhi):

   Dose same as above for checking abscess.

5. Along with any of the above.

   Tab Gasex (Himalaya):

   2 to 3 tablets be taken thrice to check stomach inflammetion, burning sensation etc.

6. Treatment should continue for long time.

7. To check temperature rising due to abscess.

Pranda Syrup (Baidyanath) 2 teaspoonful thrice daily or 4 (*four*) hourly till high temperature falls.

PEPTIC ULCER

Peptic ulcer is also called as *Gastric Ulcer* since the formation of the ulcer is due to the combined action of the over production of hydrochloric acid and pepsin—an important digestive enzyme. The ulcer is formed when the enzyme attempts to absorb the hydrochloric acid and in this effort the mucus lining of the stomach wall—called *Intestinal Mucosa*—is burnt. What becomes of the burnt area is a troublesome wound or gastric ulcer. Peptic ulcer is the common name of gastric ulcer and duodenal ulcer.

The important feature of the presence of ulcer in stomach is the irritating and burning sensation, intense pain with or without food. Epigastric pain, vomiting tendency, indigestion, vomiting of blood, blood in stool and sweating during the rise of pain are some features that needs thorough tests and checks to detect an ulcer.

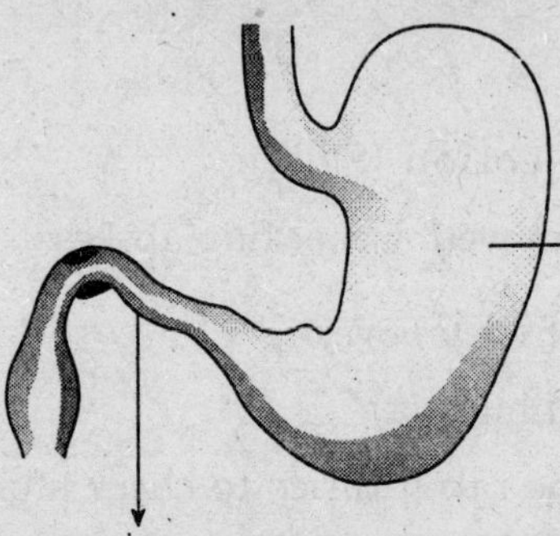

Note: In most cases of pyloric stenosis, surgery is done in the long run but in Homeopathy the combined drugs **Hydrastis 1x, Condurango 3x, Carbo Veg 3x** taken after one hour after meal improves this case.

Treatment

1. Firstly Barium-meal X-ray should be done to confirm the presence of ulcer, the size of ulcer and the part where it is formed.
2. Stool test and gastroscopy may be required depending upon the doctor's decision.
3. Absolute non-spiced food and cold (not hot) drinks are suitable. Liquid rice with milk or curd is best.
4. To treat ulcer the medicines usually helpful are:
   a) Antacids such as **Robina 1x** need to be administered.
   b) **Aristolochia 1x, Euphorbum 3x,** or **Hydrastin Mur 3x** and **Mimosa Pudica 1x** (all mixed up) taken 1 (*one*) hour after food or **Asclepias incarnata 1x, Nigella Sativa 1x, Sal China 1x, Negyndo 1x** (all mixed up) is equally good.

c) **Ficus Religosa 1x, Dhurba 1x, Ae. India 1x** are also good in ulcers. Similarly, **Geranium Mac Q, Hammemelis Q, Symphytum 1x** (mixed up) alternately with **Uranium Nit 30** or **Arg Nit 30** relieves bleeding and pain.

d) The composition of **Babul** (*Acacia Arabica*), **Mako** (*Black Night Shade*), **Guruch** (*Tinospora Cordi*), **Kasni** (*Wild Chicory*), **Deekamali** (*Gardenia Gummi*). Boiled and then 10 ml taken thrice daily.

e) To get relief from gastritis acompanying ulcer the composition of **Sengha namak** (*Sodium Cloridum*), **Kalanamak** (*Black Salt*) and **Amla** (*Embilica Officinelis*) all chewed in small dose in powder form. Preferably adding **Sap of Bot trees** (*Ficus— Bengalanese*) or **Dhurva** (*Cynadon D*).

Patent Ayurvedic Medicines

1. **Styplon Tablet** (Himalaya):

   2 tablets 4 (*four*) hourly to check ulcer bleeding, if any.

or

2. **Posex Forte Tablet** (Charak):

   2 tablets 4 (*four*) hourly to check ulcer bleeding.

3. **Gasex Tablet** (Himalaya):

   2 to 3 tablets thrice daily after food.

4. **Zyme Tablet** (Zandu):

   Same as above to check burning sensation, acidity, flatulence etc.

5. **Soolantak Capsule** (Garg):

   1 to 2 capsules with lukewarm water to check pain.

4

6. **Shool Kesari Injection** (Mishra):

   1 injection once or twice daily as required for controlling pain.

7. **Shoolbarjini Bati** (Baidyanath):

   2 tablets 4 (*four*) hourly to check pain.

POISONS AND ACIDS

In case a person drinks poison or acid—knowingly or unknowingly—the following treatment should be given:

A. **Acid Poisoning:** The symptom of burning in the throat, thirst, blood vomiting, etc. are seen. Any type of acid it be:

   1. No stomach wash.
   2. **Charcoal powder** mixed with water be given to drink or **Soda bicarb** mixed with water, orally or through stomach tube.
   3. **Opium 6** or **Belladona 6x** internally 5 times a day.
   4. Saline/oxygen as necessary. Lime water in moderate dose be given (1 cup to 1/2 glass) depending on the quantity of acid taken.

B. **Barbiturate Poisoning:** Due to barbiturate intake the patient often has respiratory problems, cyanosis and hypotension. The patient in due course feels sleepy and becomes unconscious.

   In such cases stomach wash is necessary if the poison is not vomited out completely. Charcoal powder with water can also be given. **Natrum Sulph 3x** (5 to 10 tablets) with water be given. Oxygen, saline be given as required. For respiratory failure, hypotension etc. treatment accordingly be done.

C. **Cannabis Indica** (Ganja): This is a poisonous plant. used extensively as an intoxicating substance by the addicts. But excess intake may prove fatal. The action of this poison is manifested by symptoms of excess laughing, talking, twitching and contraction of body. Physical weakness, rapid pulse initially, then deep sleep or unconsciousness, that may lead to death.

To counter the poison **Mag Sulph 6x, Strychnea Phos 6,** or slaked lime water or tamarind water be given. Later **Arsenic 30, Carbo-veg 30** may be essential.

D. **Carbondioxide:** If any person is affected by spurious gases, he should be immediately taken to fresh air. water be sprinkled on him. Symptoms of vomiting, muscular incoordination, contraction, loss of senses etc. may be noticed. If heart beat is slowing down then **Adrenalin 6x** be administered, if senseless, then coramine be administered or simultaneously if the person is able to drink hot milk with 3 teaspoonful of wine/brandy be given.

In the non-availability of the above medicines, **Arsenic 30, Carbo-veg 30** or **Camphor 30, Belladona 30, Cadmium Sulph 30** according to symptom becomes necessary.

E. **Cyanide Poisoning:** In this case very few persons survive. Immediately after Cyanide intake Cyanosis and respiratory failure starts. To encounter it give **Natrum Nitricum 6x** or **Atropia 6x** frequently followed by inhalation of **Amyl Nitrate 1x.** After overcoming the crisis **Mag Sulph 6x/6** be given (*Kali Carb* 6x and *Ferrus Sulph* 6x) can also be used as antidote.

F. **DDT and TIK 20 Poisoning:** These are deadly insecticides. If somebody drinks any of the two knowingly or unknowingly, then symptoms of vomiting, muscular twitching, burning sensation, high pulse beat, then slowing down of pulse as condition becomes serious, loss of senses etc. finally death. Stomach wash with **Mag-Sulph 3x** and **Mag Sulph/Atropia Sulph 6x** internally and on the basis of symptoms treatment be done

G. **Kerosene Poisoning:** The symptoms are kerosene smell from mouth; there may or may not be vomiting, pulse will become slow and patient would gradually become unconscious—all depending upon the quantity of kerosene intake.

In this case:

1. Liquid paraffin should be given to the patient to drink. Stool and vomiting be allowed.
2. No stomach wash.
3. **Atropia Sulph 6x** internally 5 times a day. Oxygen and saline, if necessary.
4. Later **Natrum Sulph 6x,** internally, if necessary thrice a day.
5. There can be pain and burning sensation in the mouth and stomach and even bluishness of skin in extreme cases. So, treatment must follow according to symptoms. To avoid risk administer **Mag-Sulph 6x** frequently.

H. **Opium Poisoning:** The symptoms are sleepiness, contraction of pupil, pulse feeble and body cold. Injection Lethidrone as antidote. Dextrose and oxygen may be necessary. Stomach wash is necessary or vomiting be induced, then **Atropia 6** be given, **Coffea 6x, Hing** (*Asafoetida* 6x) to neutralise opium toxins, milk mixed with butter be given to neutralise the opium action. If pulse, heart beat slows or body turns blue give **Adrenaline 6x.**

I. **Overdose of Dititalis Poisoning:** Due to overdose of digital is, patient can die due to cardiac arrest. Slow pulse, unconsciousness, heart block are seen. To counter it **Kali Mur 3x** with water or **Kali Mur 6** on tongue be given. **Carbo-veg 6x** to overcome senselessness, also **Coffea 6x** and **Atropia 6x** to normalise pulse rate.

J. **Phenol Poisoning:** In case phenol is taken, stomach wash should be immediately done or charcoal powder with water administered. **Magnesium Sulph 1x** or **3x** with water several times a day, dose depending on the severity of the case. Abdominal pain, diarrhea, vomiting and collapse are the symptom. So, accordingly, treatment should be done. For relieving of pain **Morphia 6** may be necessary.

K. **Spurious Alcohol Poisoning:** In case of spurious alcohol drunk, stomach wash is necessary. **Sodium bicarb** with water be administered. For symptoms of vomiting, hypotension or hypoglycemia treatment accordingly be done—**Cuprum Ars 6** and **Belladona 6** alternately.

or

Cumphor 6, Coffea 6 alternately, **Strychnia Phos 6** also be given in place of coffea or incurrently.

The mixture of **Dhania** (*Corriander*) **IMLI** (*Tamarind*) be given with water time to time as home remedy.

L. **Strammonium Poisoning:** The symptoms are diluted pupil, mouth dry, delirium, blurred vision, tachycardia. Stomach wash necessary or administer charcoal powder mixed in water to delay absorption of poison or start lavage with magnesium sulfate diluted in water in the ratio of 10 g : 100 ml of water. In case of high fever and other problems treat accordingly.

Homeopathic Pilocarpin 6x and **Caffine 6x** be given. The juice of **Brinjal leaves** or **Sankpuspi** (*Canscora decusata*) can be administered as home remedy.

M. **Other types of Poisoning:** If other poisons such as Tik 20 or any pest killing chemicals are taken, then charcoal powder with water be administered or soda bicarb. with water be given.

For spasms, breathing trouble, treatment as required be done. Stomach wash should be tried first. **Atropia Sulph 6x** or **Magnesium Sulph 6x** be given 4 to 5 times a day or more as may be the requirement.

PYORRHEA (ASSOCIATED CASE)

Pyorrhea is a wound or ulcer of the teeth and the gum, pus is formed as in any wound and spread to the surrounding teeth and gum. So intense pain, swelling of gum and tongue with foul smell coming from mouth is the common symptom. Bacterial infection is generally noticed. To prevent pyorrhea proper care of teeth is essential. Pyorrhea leads to gastro-intestinal disorders.

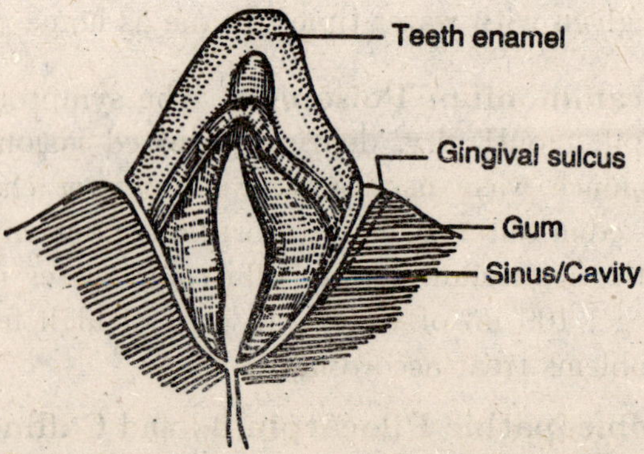

Cavity or Sinus formation in tooth harbours Pus Bacterial infection resulting in the disease of pyorrhea.

Treatement

1. To check pus and fissures use internally **Arsenic-Iod 30** and **Kreosotum 3x** and **Cistus 3x** (*mixed*) externally, also **Kreosotum 6** internally is effective.

or

2. **Acid Carb 200**, or **Euphorbum 6**, or **Acetea Spicata 6** internally and **Cistus 3x/Staphisgria 1x** externally.
3. Even **Aconite** and **Tarentula Cub 200** (*combined*) taken internally cures pain. **Myristica Sebi 3x** is also effective.
4. In extreme cases **Tellurium 6, Cal Picric 30** are effective.
5. The Sap of **Banyan twigs** (*Ficus religosa*), **Thuhar** (*common milk hedge/Euphorbia*) and clove oil mixed and externally applied to relieve pain and pus also powder of **Babul** (*Acacia Arabica*), **Kanghi Booti** (*country Mallow/Abilabutelon Indicum*) or **Siris bark** (*Albizzia Odoratissima*) or **Deekamali** (*Gardenia-Gummfera*) mixed with **Seasum Oil** be applied externally or decoction prepared without adding seasum oil be taken internally or Juice of **Gauma Booti** (*Leucas Caphalotes*) externally and its decoction internally in 5 ml dose.

Patent Ayurvedic Medicines

1. **Kapina Tablet** (Himalaya):

   1 to 2 tablets thrice daily with lukewarm water.

2. **Gumtone Tooth Powder** (Charak):

   For local application thrice daily.

3. **Karamati Tablet** (Rajbaid Sitalprasad):

   2 tablets thrice daily with lukewarm water for some days.

TUBERCULOUS PERITONITIS

It is the peritonitis caused by the migration of tuberculosis bacteria from the tuberculosis disease of any of the organs surrounding the abdomen or the peritoneum. Tuberculosis of the intestine, hernia, genitals, uterus, even lungs.

In this type of peritonitis fever, abdomial pain at the site of the disease, loss of weight and investigation may reveal encysted fluid containing pus and blood. Bariam-meal X-ray can also detect tuberculous lesion with mantoux and AFB tests show positive result.

Treatment

1. Drainage of the intestinal fluid or drying up if less, and if possible.

2. Treatment of general tuberculosis should be done.

3. In general **Tuberculinum 200**, or **Chloromycetin 30, Senecio 6, Plumbum 6, Anthraxin 200, Borax 30** are used. (*Phytolecca* 6x, *Hammamelis* 6x) combined alternately with **Tuberculinum** or **Anthraxin** or **Chloromycetin** are important treatment. In general **Geranum Mac 1x, Symphytom 1x** and **Arsenic A 12x** 4 (*four*) hourly give good result. Later increase the gap and introduce **Cal. Phos 12x** twice daily.

4. The composition of **Guruch** (*Tinospora Cordi*), **Parvar** (*Trichosanthes Dioica*), **Babul** (*Acacia Arabi*), **Mako** (*Black Night Shade*), **Kasni** (*Wild Chicory*). Boiled and cooled and 10 ml thrice daily.

Another composition with **Babul** (*Acacia Arabica*), **Kukraunda** (*Blumea Lacera*), **Shesam** (*Dalbergia Sissoo*), **Haritki** (*Termenalia Chebbula*). 10 ml of Decoction 3 to 4 times daily. This composition will cure inflammation as well as infection if any.

Patent Ayurvedic Medicines

1. **Special T.B. Injection** (Bundelkhand):

   1 to 2 ml regularly or alternative days.

2. **Bakeri Tablet** (Zandu):

   3 to 4 tablets thrice daily to check T.B.

3. **Kortina Tablet** (Charak):

   2 to 3 tablets thrice daily for checking T.B.

   With any of the above treatment give:

4. **Shoolbarjini Bati** (Baidyanath):

   1 to 2 tablets thrice daily to check pain.

5. **Bolbadh Ras** (Baidyanath):

   If necessary 1 to 2 tablets to check internal bleeding.

6. **Pranda Syrup** (Baidyanath):

   1 to 2 teaspoonful thrice daily to check high temperature.

7. Treatments to continue for a long time; after recovery give syrup A.G. Forte (*Deccan Ayurvedic*)—it is a restorative tonic.

TYPHOID AND PARA-TYPHOID FEVER

Typhoid and para-typhoid fever is called the *Enteric fever.* It is due to the reason that the bacterias *salmonella typhi* and *para-typhi* both infect and inflame the human small intestine, upsetting the intestinal function and causing even ulcers and rigidity of intestinal muscles and the toxins released in the blood causes fever which is high and rises gradually.

Loose stool, bilious or green coloured, vomiting tendency, abdominal discomfort with pain and rigidity, enlargement of spleen even liver with ascending fever calls for immediate treatment.

White tongue with reddish edges, cracks on tongue, red eyes and great weakness also help in diagnosis of this bad disease.

Blood test, stool and urine test etc. may be done to confirm the disease.

Bed rest and glucose water, later light food is necessary till recovery. It must be noted that typhoid fever is not a fever, it is a symptom only, hence medicine to suppress the fever should never be used unless there is hyperthermia or fever rising above 40.5°C (105°F) The cure of the intestinal disease would automatically bring down the fever.

Treatment

1. Typhoidinum 30 or Chloromycetin 30 or Acid Mur 200 alternately with a mixture of hydrastic 1x, Baptisa 1x or Echinesca 1x. Terebinth 30 may be given in lower abdomen bloating or uneasiness.

2. Paronichia illice 1x, Acacia Arabica 1x are also good.

3. For other Naturopath practitioners the composition of Guruch (*Tinospora Cordi*), Pokhar Mul (*Inula Racemosa*), Kantakari (*Solanom Xantho*), Babul (*Acacia A*) boiled and 10 ml thrice daily or standard drugs such as Praneshwar Rasa or Sauvagyabati.

or

4. The composition of Khaksi (*Sisymbrium Irio*), Karanjwa (*Caesalpina Bondu*), Mako (*Black Night Shade*) decoction of these be given along with Clax of stag's horn, 10 ml thrice daily.

5. For green coloured watery stool Elaterium 6, Mercurius Dulchis 6.

or

6. Effective medicine to tone up both liver and spleen etc. be given. Refer chapter on Jaudice.

Patent Ayurvedic Medicines

1. **Jawar Sanghar Capsule** (Mishra):

   1 or 2 capsules twice daily or 6 (*six*) hourly to check both high temperature and stomach inflammation.

2. **Poxes Forte Tab** (Charak):

   2 tablets 4 (*four*) hourly to check bleeding if any.

3. **Shoolbarjini Bati** (Baidyanath):

   2 tablets 4 (*four*) hourly to check intestinal spasm and pain.

4. **Sidhika Dastona** (Sidhi):

   2 tablets thrice daily effective in gastrointestine with or without fever.

5. Later Laxative as **Regulax Forte Tab** (Charak) or **Herbolax** (Himalaya):

   May be taken if necessary.

6. After recovery **A.G. Forte Syrup** (Deccan Āyurvedic):

   Should be taken to regain health and energy.

7. If necessary **Gasex Tablet** (Himalaya):

   2 tablets twice daily may be given 1/2 (*half*) hour after meal along with treatment 1.

VOMITING

Vomiting is a common symptom of gastro-entero disorder faced by most of the people. Since it is natural for the body to refuse all that is poisonous if the food taken is poisonous, or spurious, or any other chemical and mineral substances, such as acids, be taken, then the irritation caused in the stomach is immediately signalled to the brain, which in association with the hypothalamas and the nervous system contracts the diaphragm, the intestine and the abdominal muscles. By this contraction the spurious substance is expelled from the stomach, contraction leads to vomiting.

In general vomiting is caused by gastro-entero tract injury, inflammation, infections, ulcers, cancer, presence of tumour and fetus, allergy and cerebral injury, migraine, drugs etc.

If vomiting is not immediately stopped after one or two vomiting bouts, then dehydration may lead to collapse and even death.

The successful medicines are the one which can block the dopamine receptors in the chemoreceptor trigger zone.

Treatment

1. Vomiting caused by indigestion—a mixture of **Carbo-veg 6x, Ipecac 6x** and **China 6x** 10 drops in 15 to 30 minutes gap.

2. To reduce tension, inflammations, irritation of stomach generally present during vomiting a mixture of **Aconite 6** and **Apis mel 6** or **Arsenic 6** and **Belladona 6**, 3 to 5 drops incurrently.

3. If vomiting is so severe that nothing remain in stomach, even water given is vomited out, then 10 drops of mixture of **Gaultheria 6x, Ipecac 6x** and **Mag Phos 12x** be given. Even **Amygdalus Pers 6x** is effective.

4. If infection is doubted then treatment 3, be followed by **Arsenic Sulph 6,** or **Sulphur 30,** or **Cuprum Ars 6.** So treatment 3 and 4 alternatively is best to relieve pain, spasm and vomiting.

5. If vomiting does not subside then the mixture of **Elaterian 6, Ipecac 6x, Mag Phos 12x** (*tablet*) also mixed up, followed by a dose of opium 30 in 1 (*one*) hour gap. These are vomiting cases, general and infection related, that the above medicines can cure. But for vomiting cases induced by poison, e.g., Tic 20, acids, cancer, ulcer, cerebral injury etc. specific treatment and first-aid for these type of cases should be done and vomiting should be allowed for few bouts and then only checked.

Patent Ayurvedic Medicines

1. **Vomitone Tablet** (Charak):

   1 tablet 1/2 (*half*) hourly or as required.

2. **Pet Gasnasak Capsules** (New India Ayurvedic):

   1 capsule twice daily.

3. **Gasex Tablet** (Himalaya):

   2 tablets 1 (*one*) hourly in serious cases.

4. **Alsarex Tablet** (Charak):

   2 tablets thrice or 4 (*four*) hourly as required in bileous vomiting flatulance etc.

5. **Gastrodap Tablet** (Deccan Ayurvedic):

   2 tablets with lukewarm water as required.

6. **Kalyan Sundar Injection** (Bundelkhand):

   1 ml twice daily 1/2 ml for children and 1/4 ml for infants.

WORMS

The different types of worms finding a breeding place in the human intestines are:

Round worm, Hookworm, Thread worm, Tape worm, Pin worm, Whip worm etc.

These worm causes a lot of stomach problems line nausea, vomiting, dyspepsia, dysentery, intestinal bleeding, anemia, intestinal obstruction etc., all of which may turn fatal and even cause death.

Treatment

The extracts of **Vidangha** (*Embelia Ribes*), **Seed of Palash** (*Butea Frondosa*) and **Bark of Neem** (*Azadirachta Indica*) in mixed form be administered twice daily also the root of **Anar** (*Pomegranate*), **Babchi** (*Psorales-Corylifolia*) be boiled and decoction taken twice daily. Another decoction of **Karer** (*Capparis Decidua*), **Katai Chhoti** (*Solanum Xantho*) and **Nim** is helpful in expelling worms.

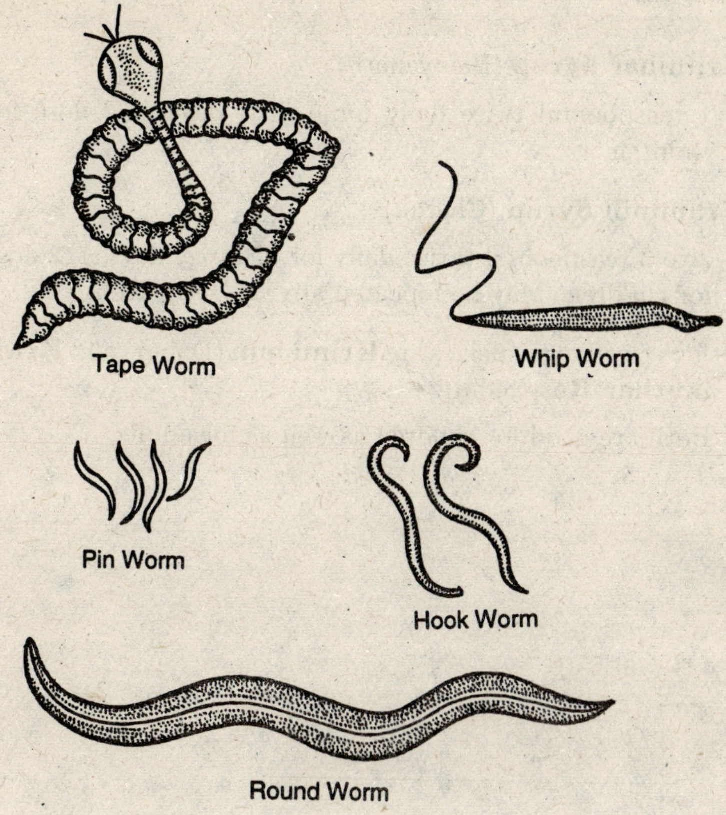

Some types of intestinal worms.

In Homeopathy, **Cina 30, Santonin 1x** are for pin and round worms. **Chelone Q** is for all types of worms **Filix Mas 1x** is for Tape worm. **Embelia Rebes Q** is for pin, round and hook worms. **Chelone** or **Filix Mas** (10–15 drops) with lukewarm water taken in empty stomach everyday, not more than twice daily. For hook-worm specifically **Thymol 6x** is used. **Teucrium 6x** for Pin worms. However, nowadays Tab **Membendazole** is used effectively for all types of worms.

Patent Ayurvedic Medicines

1. **Krimihar Syrup** (Baidyanath):

   1 teaspoonful twice daily for 6 (*six*) days, 1/2 dose for children.

2. **Cruminill Syrup** (Charak):

   2 to 3 teaspoonful thrice daily for 3 (*three*) days, 1/2 dose for children. May be repeated after 2 (*two*) weeks.

3. Other selective medicines are **Krimi hun** (Dabur) and **Krimikuthar Ras** (Sidhi):

   Both are good for children as well as for adults.

Section II

Addresses of Some Patent Ayurvedic Medicine Producing Companies

1. **Baidyanath Ayurved Bhavan Ltd.:**

   Great Nagpur Road, Nagpur 9.

2. **Bundelkhand Ayurvedic Pharmaceutical Works:**

   Manik Chowk, Jhansi 284 009.

3. **Charak Pharmaceuticals:**

   Evergreen Industrial Estate, Bombay 400 011.

4. **Deccan Ayurvedic Pharmacy Ltd.:**

   Saidabad, Hyderabad, Andhra Pradesh.

5. **Indo-German Pharmaceuticals:**

   Lal Bahadur Shastri Marg, Bombay 83.

6. **Mishra Ayurvedic Pharmacy:**

   Jhansi, (U.P.)

7. **Martand Pharmaceuticals:**

   Post Box No. 9, Merrut 250 611.

8. **Rajbaid Sitalprasad and Sons:**

   4771 Bharat Ram Road, Dariaganj, New Delhi 2.

9. **Sri Dhanwantari Ayurvedic Pharmacy:**

   277 East Mohannagar, Amritsar, Punjab.

10. Siddhi Pharmaceutical Works:

Lalitpur, Jhansi (U.P.)

11. The Himalaya Drug Co. Ltd.:

Shivsagar, Dr. Annie Besant Road, Bombay 400 018.

12. Zandu Pharmaceuticals Works Ltd.:

Gokhale Road, Dadar, Bombay 400 025.

Medicinal Plants and Useful Parts

Adusa — *All parts.*

Amaltas — *Seed, Bark, Root.*

Amla — *Fruit.*

Anantamool — *Root.*

Apamarg — *All parts.*

Aparajita — *Seed, Fruit..*

Aroud — *Root, Leaves.*

Babul — *Bark, Gum, Leaves.*

Baibidang — *Fruit.*

Bakayan — *Bark, Leaves.*

Barun — *Root, Bark, Leaves.*

Bathua — *Seed, Stem.*

Bavchi — *Seed.*

Bidarikand — *Stem.*

Chirata — *Stem, Leaves.*

Daruhaldi — *Root, Bark.*

Gorakmundi — *Root, Stem.*

Gritkumari — *Leaves.*

Haritki — *Seed, Fruit.*

Indrayan — *Fruit, Flower.*

Kalmegh — *All parts.*

Kasaundi — *Leaves, Root, Seed.*

Kasni — *Seed, Leaves, Root.*

Kesar — *Seed, Flower.*

Khubkala — *Seed.*

Kutz — *Seed, Bark.*

Methi — *Seed.*

Mulhati — *Seed.*

Nagarmotha — *Root, Leaves.*

Nagkesar — *Fruit, Flower, Stem.*

Pitpapada — *All parts.*

Pudina — *All parts.*

Sankpuspi — *All parts.*

Sarpanka — *Root.*

Saptaparna — *Bark, Flower.*

Satyanasi — *Root, Seed.*

Senna — *Leaves, Fruit.*

Sonapata — *Bark, Root.*

Tulsi — *Leave, Root.*

Other Household Ingredients

Elaichi — *the Ingredient itself.*

Haldi — *the Ingredient itself.*

Khaskhas (opium seed) — *the Ingredient itself.*

Lahsun — *the Ingredient itself.*

Lovng — *the Ingredient itself.*

Saunth — *the Ingredient itself.*

Sounf — *the Ingredient itself.*

Zeera (black) — *the Ingredient itself.*

Zeera (white) — *the Ingredient itself.*

Some Ayurvedic Medicinal Plants and Cures

ACALYPHA INDICA *(Muktajhuri)*

This drug in small quantity is helpful in diarrhea or dysentery, where there is passing of mucus or blood with stool. Heat and burning sensation in stomach, ulcer that bleed and even in blood vomit. This drug works better if given along with Sankhyapuspi (*Coxbolvulus Pluricarilis*).

ACHYRANTHES ASPERA *(Apamarga)*

This drug has the characteristics to fight infection, hence, should be useful in infective stomach problems such as hepatitis, dysentery, diarrhea, even in cases of stomach ulcer and appendicitis. It is preferred in cholera if administered with Acalypha Indica or Taphrasia Purpurea.

ANDROGRAPHIS PANICULATA *(Kalmegh)*

This is a popular and effective drug in checking acute or chronic stomach diseases, jaundice, liver inflammation, hepatitis, cirrhosis of liver, indigestion and lack of appetite. It is also effective in expelling worms. This drug should be preferably taken half cup empty stomach in early morning.

ARISTOLOCHIO INDICA *(Iswarmul)*

This drug is not very powerful, but has the properties to check dysentery and bloody stool, cramps and distention in stomach. It is helpful in infective stomach problems or stomach problems arising due to intake of spurious food.

ASPARAGUS RACEMOSA *(Satavari)*

This drug is helpful in jaundiced liver, burning sensation in stomach and indigestion, it regulates bile secretion and also effective in simple dropsy cases. If can be used along with (*Sarphanka*) Taphrasia Purpurea or (*Varani Khand*) Tracca Aspera to check infective stomach cases such as dysentery and diarrhea.

ATISTA RADIX *(Ashseora)*

This drug is generally used in all types of acute and chronic dysentery and diarrhea, where there is mucus blood in the stool and violent cramps in the abdomen. Once the stomach ailment is cured this drug—after a short time use—promotes digestion.

BALSAMODENDRON MUKUL *(Goggul)*

In the preparation of a variety of Naturopathic or Ayurvedic drugs the use of goggul is common. It is becasue of its reputation in increasing appetite, weakness of digestive system, infection and inflammation of stomach, flatulence and colic. It is also good as a milk diuretic, so helpful in dropsy cases.

BLUMEA ODORATA *(Kuksima)*

This drug is helpful in all bleeding cases such as blood vomiting, ulcer bleeding, bleeding piles or blood dysentery. It also has the properties to check liver inflammation and gastritis. It works better if given along with Nagkesar (*Cobras Saffron*) and Saunf (*Aniseed*).

BOERHAVIA DIFFUSA *(Purnarnava)*

This drug is reputed in checking any type of dropsy of the body, hence it is useful in all sorts of hepatic problems, jaundice and cirrhosis of liver. It is also effective in infective cases including preliminary stage of appendicitis. It also increases appetite, promotes digestion and so improves health. For better result it should be used with andrographis paniculata.

CAESALPINIA BONDUCELLA *(Karanjawa)*

This drug is effective in all infective cases, where fever is a symptom. Hepatitis, liver pain, abscess, food poison and even bacterial infection of stomach leading to stool. It works well if added with Aparajita (*Clitoria Tesnalia*) and Khubkala (*Sisymbrium Irio*).

CUMINUM CYMINUM *(Safed Zeera)*

Zeera is a very common spice, it is available in every house kitchen. It is carminative, cooling and digestive to stomach. In cases of bowel disorders, colic, diarrhea, eructation, epigastric discomfort and flatulence it is commonly used. For better result use it with corriander, ginger and aniseed.

CYPARUS SCARIOSUS *(Nagarmotha)*

This drug is helpful to tone up the digestive system, regulate the digestive secretion and good in checking stomach and abdominal inflammation. In cases of sluggish liver activity and liver pain use it, preferably with Baberang (*Embelia Ribes*).

EMBELIA RIBES *(Baberang)*

This drug is commonly applied in stomach upsets, indigestion, flatulence, intermittent diarrhea and dysentery where the presence of worms is suspected. Feeling of hunger or no appetite at all, disturbance of sleep due to worms, calls for its use. For better result use it along with Kalmegh (*Andrographis Paniculata*).

FUMARIA PARVIFLORA *(Pitpapada)*

Pitpapada is common with Ayurvedic druggists. It is generally used to increase appetite, decrease abdominal tension, eructation, epigastric tightness and dyspepsia and in all inflammatory condition of stomach where pain is a symptom. It also checks hepatic disorders and so beneficial in jaundice. For better effect use it along with Sarpankha (*Tephrosia P*).

HYDROCOTYLE ASIATICA *(Thankuni)*

Hydrocotyle is common among the general people. Most people use it as a remedy to check dysentery, but most people do not know that it is efficient in checking hepatic disorders and jaundice. In cirrhosis of liver and dropsy cases it works wonder if used with Punarnava and Kalmegh.

PISTACIA LENTISCUS *(Rumi Mastgi)*

This drug is efficient in controlling digestive disorders. All inflammation of liver, spleen etc. and also flatulence is checked by its use. In blood vomiting or gum bleeding its use is helpful. It also tones up the digestive system and checks dropsy.

PLUMBAGO ZEYLANICA *(Chitrak)*

This drug is very efficient in treating infective hepatitis and other infective stomach problems. It increases digestive capacity, checks inflammation of liver, spleen, pancreas and related fever. It should better be used along with Tephrosia P.

POLYGONUM AVICULRA *(Anjuvar)*

This drug has proved to be efficient in checking different types of bleeding including bleeding from stomach, intestine and piles. It is also effective in indigestion. Burning sensation in stomach and worms. It works well if used with Sonth (*Zingiber Officinale*) and Goggul (*Balbamodendron Mukul*).

PRUNUS COMMUNIS *(Alu Bokhara)*

The importance of this drug is in its ability to break and expel gallstone and renal stones. Besides this it is applicable in the treatment of general stomach disorders, it increases digestion and promotes health. It is also blood purifier and so checks the skin diseases, dries up both internal and external wounds and ulcer.

SAXIFRAGA LIGULATA *(Pashanved)*

In problems associated with the presence of stone, burning sensation in stomach, indigestion and chronic constipation Pashanved should be used. It regulates the body temperature by producing sweats, expelling urine and stool. Its use along with saunf (*Aniseed*) is helpful in all the above problems.

SISYMBRIUM IRIO *(Khubkala)*

Khubkala is used both by the Ayurvedic and Unnani Practitioners. It is efficient in increasing appetite and toning up of the digestive system. In chronic stomach problems with excess bile formation or excess acid formation, which leads to untimely, irregular stool and if, along with these problems, a slight rise of temperature or dryness of skin is noticed then Khubkala should be used with Goggul and Haritki.

TRINGONELA F. GRAECUM *(Methi)*

It is a household common remedy in reducing inflammation of stomach, loose stools, burning sensation in stomach, vomiting urge. In the inflammation of piles it can be used. It increases appetite, decreases flatulence and thereby regulates the body temperature. For better result use it along with Ginger and Aniseed.

1. To check sudden or acute stomach pain take 1 teaspoonful each of turmeric power, aniseed and a pinch of salt and drink with a glass of water.

2. To check sudden or acute dyspepsia problems take 1 teaspoonful each of Ajowan, Aniseed, Zeera (*common seed*) and 1/3 teaspoonful of Kali Zeera (*Black Cummin*) and a little of ginger chewed well and taken with water.

3. To check urge to vomit or vomiting, use one teaspoonful of aniseed, onion juice and two pieces of kali mirch (*Piper Nigrun*) should be chewed and taken with water.

4. To overcome constipation take 1 teaspoonful or 2 teaspoonful of Haritki power (*Termenalia chebula*) with one cup of plain water, then after one minuite take a glass of lukewarm water, this would clear the bowels.

5. To check sudden blood vomiting take 10 drops of Sandal wood (*Santalum Album*) oil, 20 drops of the extracts of Dhurba (*Cynodon Dactylom*) diluted with cold water taken at 2 (*two*) hours interval till the bleeding is checked. In place of the above even the white milky sap of Aswatha tree (*Ficus Religosa*) around 10 drops diluted with a cup of water should be taken.

6. To check the severity of Peritonitis—which generally proves fatal—prepare a powder of Haritki (*Termenalia Chebula*), Kali Mirch (*Piper Nigrum*) and add one teaspoonful of onion extract and take all these together with lukewarm water every 2 (*two*) hourly basis. If time allows and if Sarpankha (*Tephrasia purpurea*) and Rakta Sal Muli (*Bombax Malabaricum*) root or extracts can be had from Ayurved Drug Shop, they should be boiled in case of roots but not in case of powder. 2 teaspoonful of each added with the above ingredients leaving out onion juice should be administered for effective results.

TRINGONELLA UNEATA *(Ikkolul Malik)*

This drug is not very widely used but it has the properties to check stomach pain, liver pain, and inflammation and enlargement of the digestive organs such as liver, spleen, pancreas etc. In gallbladder abnormality and pain in stomach it can be used. It can expel the stones and promote proper secretive action.

Some Important Ayurvedic Remedies

1. Dyspepsia, indigestion, excessive bile secretion, sour eructation, stomach pain due to gas—*Kapdark Vashma.*

2. In case of liver malfluctioning, gallbladder stone, liver abscess, renal stone, spleen enlargement and also bleeding in stomach—*Akik Vashma.*

3. In case of jaundice liver affection and to promote blood formation—*Kasis Vashma* or *Jaundisal Syrup.*

4. In all sorts of stomach bleeding—*Kaharva* or *Bolbadh Rasa.*

5. To increase blood and correct anemia—*Kantloha Vashma.*

6. To combat constipation—*Kabz Har.*

7. To combat bleeding piles—*Pairayeed Tablet* or *Pranda Gutika.*

8. To get relief from gastritis or gas accumulation in bowels—*Gasantak Bati.*

9. To check swelling of gum, toothache, pyorrhea—*Dant Veshtari Ointment.*

10. To check dysentery and diarrhea with or without mucus and blood—*Kutzavleha* or *Bilvadi Churna.*

11. To regulate the digestive system by correcting habitual constipation—*Panchsakar Churna.*

12. To clear intestinal worms—*Vidangsav/Kirmikutar Rasa.*

13. To check fluid collection or case of dropsy—*Purnavarista* or *Dhugda Bati.*

14. In children disease with liver and spleen disorder anemia, flatulence, constipation—*Kumar Asav no. 3.*

15. To check piles, fistula and abscess—*Saptavinsati Goggul* (internally).

16. To improve digestion, purify blood, correct skin diseases frequent urine, fistula, semen loss, chronic constipation and gas accumulation—*Yogray Goggul.*

17. To check all types of abdominal pain—*Shoolbarjini Bati.*

18. To combat indigestion, flatulence, pain and increase digestive powder—*Mahasankya Bati/Raj Bati.*

19. To cure hyperacidity and gastric ulcer—*Abhipattikar Churna.*

20. To cure intestinal tuberculosis even in typhoid—*Babul arista.*

21. To combat liver and spleen problems and loss of physical development—*Yakritplihari loha.*

22. Dialation of stomach or Hernia—*Nityanand Rasa* (All the above medicines can be had from Baidyanath Ayurved Bhavan).

Some Common Investigation of Bowel Ailments

- Barium meal x-ray.
- Blood cholesterol.
- Blood urea.
- Cholecystography.
- Elis a test for T.B.
- Endoscopy.
- Liver function test.
- Liver scan.
- Pancreatic function test
- Proctoscopy.
- Serum biluribin.
- Stool test.
- Ultrasonography of abdomen.
- Urine test for bile.
- X-ray of abdomen.

AETHUSA CYNAPIUM

Symptoms: Torpid liver resulting to indigestion specially indigestion to milk, so milk is vomited out. Other types of vomiting accompanied by inflammation of stomach throbbing pain and spasms of intestinal muscles. It is not effective in vomiting associated with food-poison or stomach ulcers. Stool test show undigested food particles and bileus stool and this calls for its application. For quick action use it alternately with **Cuprum ars 30.**

Potency: 6–30.

AGRAPHIS NUTANS

Symptoms: Useful in cases of stomach or abdominal cramps resulting from intake of cold things effective in hill diarrhea patient. Feels hungry immediately after cold bath. To promote liver activity and improve digestion and also in case of flatulence creating distress in the alimentary tract it is used. Rumbling of both wind and loose feces in the intestine and frequent loose stool call for its use. It can be used along with **Podophyllum 3x** or any other related drug.

Potency: 3x–6.

AILANTHUS GLANDULOSA

Symptoms: This drug is beneficial in cases of inflammation tendency to form abscess, ulcer or abscess and ulcer have formed in any organ of digestive system. Diarrhea arising from intake of spurious food or arising from any viral or bacterial infection call for its use. Alternately can be used with any of these drugs **pyrogen 200, terramycin 30, chloromycetin 30.**

ANTIMONIUM CHLORIDUM

Symptoms: This drugs should be remembered only in cases of chronic ulcers, wounds, gangrenous ulcers and also in cancer. To heal up the wounds, abscess and cancer cases and also to alleviate the cancer pain, this drug should be alternately tried with other known anti-ulcer or anti-cancer drugs.

Potency: 3x.

APIS MELLIFICA

Symptoms: It is a very common drug in all cases of inflammation, irritation, swelling of any organ even liver, spleen, kidney, with or without collection of serous fluid therein. Apis Mel is also good in drying up the serous fluid, so helpful in cases of edema, dropsy, in other words where there is a collection of fluid in any part, alternately to be used with **Kali Carb 6x.** In other abdominal problems, dropsy, peritonitis and feeling of burning and heat in abdomen even tongue and gums seem swollen, irritable and heavy. Abdominal muscle weakness, as a result stool comes out while urinating, stool hot and watery, involuntary. Sleepless due to heat in abdomen, swelling and burning and stinging pain in anus and piles and also lower intestine.

Potency: 3x–30.

APOCYNUM CANNABINUM

Symptoms: It is a well-known drug to combat ascites and dropsy of any particular organ or whole body. It is good in improving the function of liver, gallbladder, spleen etc. Bloated abdomen, gurgling sound of fluid in abdomen, flatulence and hence a heaviness around epigastric region need IB use. Stool watery due to fluid in intestine.

Potency: 1x–6x.

BELLADONA

Symptoms: It is one of the most important and popular medicine used by both homeopaths and allopaths. The important symptom calling for its use is biot or burning hot or constrictive pain. Belladona check excessive acid secretion, hence good in promoting digestion and ulcer pain. Any sort of contraction, constriction, pain from mouth to anus calls for its prompt use. Even diarrhea, dysentery etc. caused by spurious food or alcohol are corrected promptly by its use. In this respect it is similar to arsenic or baptisa. In severe pain the extracts of belladona (*Atropia* as *Atropia Sulph*) can be used for fast relief.

Potency: 3x–200.

BERBERIS VULGARIS

Symptoms: It is a drug well-known for improving the secretion of all glands, whether it is the saliva of the mouth or biles or insulin etc. Its use improves the functions of all the organs of the digestive system and corrects conjestion or blockage if there happens to be any with the organs., Radiating pain in the liver or gallbladder region or in the lower abdomen, even pain of piles are alleviated by its use. Constant urging to stool, torpid liver, so clay coloured stool, mucus in stool, swelling up of piles, anus sore and itches due to skin diseases—all are also some symptoms where berberis is necessary.

Potency: 1x–6.

BISMUTHUM

Symptoms: It is used to check inflammation of abdomen arising due to indigestion, hyperacidity and flatulence. Bloated stomach due to gas which lead to vomiting of food and drinks now and then calls for its use. Foul eructation and gastric pain of chronic nature are symptoms where this drug is helpful.

Potency: 1x–6.

BORAX

Symptoms: Whenever there is a tendency toward constipation, resulting to fermentation of the accumulated stool and consequent formation of gas or fermentation and irritation of the mucus lining inside resulting to stool evacuated with chunks of mucus then borax is used to calm down the inflammation and tension. Gastric pain, nausea, vomiting, colitis and swelling of any affected organ e.g., painful, swelling of appendix, then borax should be thought of. Excessive secretion of saliva, ulcers or abscess with pus also calls for its use in checking the spread of infection. It can be used alternately with pyrogen, echinesia, terramycin in checking of infection.

Potency: 6x–30.

BOTULINUM

Symptoms: It is generally useful in cases of food poisoning arising from intake of tinned foodstuff or, in other words, tin poison. After taking of tinned food if there is gastroenteritis trouble, then this drug should be used for good result.

Potency: 30–200.

BOVISTA

Symptoms: This drug works wonder in case of stomach trouble caused by taking fungus affected food or water or spurious things. Swelling of abdomen with gas, which causes cramps and pain and tightness of the abdominal muscles. Even diarrhea resulting from spurious food is cured by it. Rigidity and tightness of any organ in the abdomen—if felt—then bovista should be applied. Any other stomach problem caused by allergy also calls for its use.

Potency: 6–30.

CADMIUM SULF

Symptoms: It is a very valuable drug for the treatment of infection or ulcer related cases, such as vomiting or diarrhea due to drinking of spurious water. Also effective in ulcer related vomiting of coffee coloured or black coloured vomiting. (black or coffee colour relates to presence of blood in vomit). Again, preliminary stages of painful cancer, paralysis of the intestinal and abdominal or throat muscles due to infection, inflammation or ulcer or cancer with or without fever and constiction of esophagus, resulting in difficulty in swallowing call for its use. Similarly, due to presence of blood in stool, stool evacuated is black and foul smelling. In such type of critical cases this drug should be remembered along with other anti-hemorrhage drugs.

Potency: 6–30.

CAJUPUTUM

Symptoms: It is a common drug, generally used to check flatulence and bloating of abdomen, distention of abdomen. Feeling of constriction or blockage from mouth to rectum or any particular organ. Inflammation and infection of any abdominal organ resulting to pus cells passing out in urine and stool, so both stool and urine have very offensive smell. For any of the above problems cajuputum should be used alternately with cadmium sulf or any other suitable drug.

Potency: 1x–6.

CALCAREA ARSENICA

Symptoms: This is an important remedy in all types of infection leading to enlargement and tightness of all glands including enlargement of liver, spleen, kidney. For this sake it becomes useful in malaria, kala-azar and typhoid cases. Inflammation and severe pain of appendix or presence of small tumour or cyst also call for its use. Stomach ailment causing restlessness mean that this medicine has a chance of application. In bitter saliva, driffling of saliva or mucus, gastric pain or hyperacidity this drug proved good.

Potency: 6x–200.

CAMPHORA

Symptoms: It is a drug used to raise body temperature and pulse rate. In acute diarrhea and cholera when the patient is collapsing or becoming cold as ice, for such critical patient administering of camphora is essential. It is generally used alternately with cuprum ars or cuprum sulf.

Potency: 1x–30.

CANTHARIS

Symptoms: Whenever there is a complain of great inflammation, heat and restlessness in abdomen or a sudden urge to evacuate both urine and stool and the stool is hot, burning, full of mucus, the anus too is hot, burning seems everything would go out of the anus, then to calm down the inflammation and tension in the abdomen as well as in the body and to normalise the functions that was suddenly disturbed—cantharis is a good choice.

Potency: 6–30.

CARLSBAD

Symptoms: It is a drug that needs to be used with other drugs in the treatment of ascites, cirrhosis and inactivity of liver and related problem of indigestion, pain in abdomen, specially in liver region, also for inactivity of kidney and pancreas. To tone up the digestive organs, its use cannot be discounted.

Potency: 3x–6.

CHINA

Symptoms: It is a very valuable remedy in treatment of stomach trouble. **Flatulence,** bloating of stomach, sluggishness of liver resulting to dyspepsia, eructation of sour water, feeling of weight in stomach, severe gastric pain, gallstone pain, all these are cured by china. It has sometimes expelled **small stones** from gallbladder and proved effacious in controlling diarrhea and its resultant **physical weakness** due to fluid loss from body. For better and quick result it should be used in combination with chionanthus or berberis vul.

Potency: 1x–30.

CHOLESTERINUM

Symptoms: It is respected drug for its proven quality in treating of cancer of the liver and other digestive organs. Diminished activity of liver and gallbladder causing indigestion and presence of pain in stomach specially in the liver, gallbladder or pancreas and location of pus cells in stool accompanied by liver pain or liver abscess or ulcer in abdomen.

Potency: 3x–6.

CICUTA VIROSA

Symptoms: Its action is limited to neurological cases such as spasmodic contraction of stomach resulting in vomiting or **nervous dyspepsia, non-stop hiccough,** chocked up oeosophagus, **rigidity** in some parts of the body and rumbling **flatulence** is checked by its application.

Potency: 6–200.

CINA

Symptoms: It is a popular drug and generally used to expel worm infesting the intestine. Nausea, vomiting, heat in stomach craving for sweets call for its use and if suspected that the patient is suffering from worms then, after stool, test if presence of ova is confirmed then cina should be used.

Potency: 3x–30.

CISTUS CANADENSIS

Symptoms: This is a costly drug. It is demanded for its efficiency in curing abscess, malignant ulcers, tumour, cyst and other eruptions in the abdomen. Even swelling and inflammation of any organ such as suppurative cases as that of an acute or chronic appendix, stomach ulcers etc. can be cured by its proper use.

Potency: 1x–30.

CORNUS CIRCINATA

Symptoms: It is a drug whose sphere of action is limited to problem of liver and hepatitis, indigestion, with bloated stomach and mild constant pain in stomach, burning sensation in stomach call for its application. Clay-coloured and offensive *diarrhea with expulsion of flatus* is a indication for the choice of this drug.

Potency: 1x–6.

CROTON TIGLIUM

Symptoms: It is a remarkable drug having the properties to check diarrhea (water-like) with or without cramps in stomach immediately. Similarly, it is effective in checking vomiting. Frequent undigested stool—even with or without mucus—is cured by its application.

Potency: 6x–30.

CUPRUM ARSENITUM

Symptoms: It is a very important medicine in treatment of infective diarrhea, dysentery and accompanying violent ab dominal pain, cholera, gastro-enteritis, mucus colitis. Better results obtained if used alternately with kurvchi or croton tig etc. in diarrheal and vomiting cases. It is also used to treatment of inflammatory neurological pain.

Potency: 6x–200.

CYCLAMEN

Symptoms: It is not a very common drug but yet is known for curing violent diarrhea and vomiting, non-stop hiccough, diarrhea after tea or coffee, feeling of thirstlessness and spot pain around anus or perineum.

Potency: 6–30.

DIOSCOREA VILLOSA

Symptoms: This durg is famous as belladonna in checking of sudden *severe pain.* Violent pain, shooting, cutting pain in the abdominal muscles or in any organ, e.g., radiating and cutting pain in the gallbladder region or in iliac-fossa and pelvic region. In all sorts of clutching pain dioscorea has to be remembered. It is also well-known for checking of gas and **gastric pain,** with or without diarrhea or dysentery. It activates the digestive actions and promotes secretion of digestive juices and control amebiasis and hot diarrhea.

Potency: 1x–6.

ECHINACEA

Symptoms: It is a very reputed drug. Commonly used to fight infections, septic cases, ulcers, gangrene etc. From its characteristics it is clear that it should be applied to cure infection and septic or pyogenic related diseases. Ulcer or abscess in stomach or any other organ, even inflamed and septic stage of appendicitis, this drug is very reliable. In infective diarrhea or colitis or infected mucus dysentery such as diarrhea due to typhoid are cured by its use.

Potency: 1x–6.

ELATERIUM

Symptoms: It is a remarkable drug, its action is more striking on the digestive organs than on other organs. Violent vomiting or diarrhea, jet watery forceful with cutting and clutching in the lower or upper abdomen due to stomach infection or food poisoning or indigestion; whatever it be, if violent vomiting or diarrhea has to be checked, then elaterium is magic drug.

Potency: 6–30.

FICUS RELIGIOSA

Symptoms: It is a very effective drug used in controlling hemorrhages from any organ and of any type. For vomiting of bright red blood it is very prominent in action. Also used in treatment of mucus diarrhea, dysentery, amebiasis and ulcer of stomach. It can be used in combination with other anti-hemorrhagic drug.

Potency: 1x.

FILIX-MAS

Symptoms: Just as the drug chelone, Filix Max is a drug having specific properties to expel tape worm from the intestine. Whenever symptoms of nausea, indigestion, wind, colic etc. is noted, it can be used. In constipation too it is applicable, but its name reckoned as a anti-tape worm drug. 1x–3x (10–15) drops or, as suitable according to the age, is to be taken in early morning empty stomach and continued, if necessary, but not for long time.

Potency: 1x–3x.

FLURICUM-ACIDUM

Symptoms: This is a well-known anti-infective, antiseptic drug. It is major sphere of action is on wounds, abscess, ulcer and, in any other cases where gangrene, necrosis or tissue destruction take place, so it can be applied in ulcer of stomach, rectum etc. It is also useful in cirrhosis of liver, septic appendicitis and to correct ill-effects of drugs and alcohol, eructation and where cold things give relief, in such symptom, fluricum acidum is beneficial.

Potency: 6–200.

GAMBOGIA

Symptoms: Gambogia is specifically an anti-diarrheal drug. Jet watery diarrhea with constrictive pain around navel, stool offensive smelling with little mucus or blood, heat and burning sensation in abdomen and rectum, whatever be other symptoms, if it is diarrhea or dysentery, gambogia like croton tig should be used.

Potency: 6x–30.

GAULTHERIA

Symptoms: It is a well-known pain-killer. Muscular, neurological or bone pain, whatever be the cause of pain in acute gastric pain, liver pain, obstructive gallbladder pain, even pain of appendicitis is checked by its use. Vomiting due to gastritis is also controlled by it.

Potency: 1x–6.

GENTIANA LUTEA

Symptoms: This drug should be known to be a appetilte stimulant. It stimulates the secretion of digestive juices and corrects hepatic disorders, feeling of heaviness in stomach and eructation of salty water. It also calms the tension and uneasiness in stomach arising due to indigestion and excessive and deficient bile secretion.

Potency: 6x–6.

GERANIUM MACULATUM

Symptoms: It is a very efficient anti-hemorrhagic drug. Bleeding of any sort and occurring in any part of the body and also blood vomiting is arrested by its correct use. It is also helpful in bleeding ulcers of intestine and other found wounds and abscess. Besides these, it has properties to heal chronic offensive mucus dysentery and diarrhea and urge to go to stool every time yet very little is evacuated due to constipation. It also checks hyperacidity in stomach.

Potency: 1x–6.

HAMAMELIS VIRGINICA

Symptoms: It is a very popular drug. Its main function is to check bleeding from any part of the body and also to reduce inflammation, swelling of any organ. Bleeding from stomach, intestine, piles, soreness and tightness of liver spleen and soreness of piles and varicose and stiff veins and muscles of injured part of the body. It can be used in combination with other anti-hemorrhagic drugs.

Potency: 1x–6.

HEDEOMA

Symptoms: It is a uncommon drug in treatment of abdominal ailments. But it is known to cure ailments arising from lack of digestive juices in the stomach resulting to heaviness in stomach and formation of wind. Stomach pain before or after food with a feeling of heaviness in stomach, tearing pain in abdomen due to movement of wind are checked by its use.

Potency: 6x–6.

HYDRASTIS

Symptoms: It is a well-known drug in the treatment of general stomach disturbances, accumulation of catarrh in stomach, passing of mucus with stool or urine. Hyperacidity leading to formation of ulcer in stomach. It is also good in stimulating secrection of digestive juices and improving weight of body. Hardness and cirrhosis of liver, liver abscess, ulcer, painful and ulcerative piles, inflamed appendix, discharge of pus cells in stool are cured by its use. Constant saliva in mouth, tongue swollen and painful are curved by its use. Hydrastin Sulph 3x is used in infective ulcerative condition of bowels as in typhoid.

Potency: 1x–6.

KALI BICHROMICUM

Symptoms: Kali bichromicum is an effective drug. It is usually applied in the treatment of **chronic ulcer** in stomach and intestine. It checks to some extent the hypersecretion of bile and acid in the stomach and—by facilitating the persistaltic activity—it keeps the stomach free from the acid and biles and fermentation of undigested food. Other function of this drug is to fight the ill effects of wine and its resultant pain and cirrhosis of liver, fatty infiltration of liver, periodic bileous vomiting and dilation of stomach etc. are cured by its use.

Potency: 6–200.

KALI NITRICUM

Symptoms: It is applicable in case of gastro-enteritis inflammation and pain in abdomen. In case of diarrhea following any spurious food or food-poisoning it should be used.

In the case of malfunctioning of liver or cirrhosis of liver or painful spleen and pancreas it is helpful, also reduces the dropsy of any particular organ or the whole body. In case of suppurative appendicitis or abscess and septic cases it should be used.

Potency: 6–200.

KOUSSO

Symptoms: It is efficiently used in the expulsion of tape worm from the intestine. Nausea, vomiting, stomachache, dyspepsia etc. related to the presence of tape worm in the intestine is cured by it. 1/2 oz of this drug mixed with lukewarm water and taken empty stomach in the morning may be repeated, if requried.

Potency: 1x.

LEPTANDRA

Symptoms: This drug has a good name in Homeopathy, wherever the stomach disease relates to improper or sluggish functioning of liver, gallbladder spleen, resulting in indigestion of food, then leptandra should be remembered.

Again in rise of bilirubin in blood in jaundice and cirrhosis of liver, bileous stool and vomit, as may be the case, leptandra is essential. It is very effective if the patient complain muddy coloured stool, sour smell in body or black stool (presence of blood) and oozing of blood from anywhere in the bowels, as in typhoid cases, then laptandra should be first thought of. Even in increasing the tonacity of the bowels and rectum muscle it can be used.

Potency: 1x–6.

LIATRIS SPICATA

Symptoms: Its action is more marked on the function of liver, spleen, kidney etc. In short, whenever any of these **malfunctions** and in all types and stages of **dropsy** it should be applied.

It is also effective in ulcers and diarrhea. It is also a diuretic, so, produces more urine, cleans the kidney and consequently reduces dropsy.

Potency: 1x–6.

MAGNESIA CARBONICA

Symptoms: This drug is helpful in cases of hyperacidity, sour eructation and heaviness in the upper abdomen in the epigastric region. Better tates, bileous taste in mouth, bileous vomit, bileous stool, dyspepsia, swelling and pain in liver, gallbladder etc. It checks dysentery and diarrhea with or without mucus and blood. Liver inactive, unable to digest even milk are symptoms that call for magnesia carb. It also checks inflammation of bowels, colitis and excessive gas. Except in diarrhea and dysentery it gives better result, if used alternately with bryonia 30.

Potency: 6x–30.

MAGNESIA MURIATICA

Symptoms: It increases flow of blood in the digestive organs, hence it is effective in normalising the malfunctioning of the digestive organs. In fatty, sluggish, cirrhotic liver, gallbladder, sluggishness, lack of normal bile flow, gallbladder pain and resultant lack of digestive powder, presence of constipation, marble like stool, etc. are cured by it. Besides the above it has the other curative powders as that of magnesia carbonica.

Potency: 6–200.

MAGNESIA PHOSPHORICA

Symptoms: This drug is generally used in the treatment of neurological problems, hence, it is applicable in all sorts of pain in abdomen, even gastric pain with or without accompanying diarrhea or dysentery, eructation, hiccough, feeling of constriction, squeezing, spasm etc. are effectively cured by it. Presence of troublesome gas in lower abdomen is cured by its use. In checking diarrhea it is efficient. It should be preferably used with similar alternative drug.

Potency: 6–200.

MAGNESIA SULPHURICA

Symptoms: Magnesia sulphurica in pure form—available in market in the name of epsom salt—is a anti-constipation drug. Obstinate and chronic constipation is relieved by its use. But when taken in higher potency as 200 it checks urges for stool, dysentery and accumulation of gas in bowels. It calms down the tension in the abdomen. Bileous problem, sour eructation and gallbladder inflammation, sore-liver, dropsy, even ulcer expansion is checked by it.

Potency: 6x–200.

MENTHA PIPERITA

Symptoms: It is used in simple type of colic arising from dyspepsia and accumulation of gas. Stomach remains bloated all the time and eructation of sour water etc. are cured by it.

Potency: 1x–3x.

MERCURIUS IODATUS RUBER

Symptoms: It is a germicide and to some extent a bacteriacide drug. All types of infection related cases including stomatitis, ulcers, abscess and enlargement of glands, liver, spleen etc. are checked by it. Profuse saliva, swollen tongue, pain in throat, preliminary stage of appendicitis and even in typhoid it is useful. Discontinue its use if allergy or reaction or feeling of uneasiness is seen.

Potency: 6x–30.

MILLEFOLIUM

Symptoms: It is a noted drug for arresting various types of hemorrhages. Blood vomit, blood with stool, blood with urine, bleeding piles etc. all bleeding of bright red blood are checked by its use.

Potency: 1x–6x.

MURIATICUM ACIDUM

Symptoms: This drug is a germicide—to some extent a bactericide—so its use is seen in all infective cases as abscess, ulcers, also allergy from food, swollen tongue, gums, piles etc. are cured by it. Problems associated with drinking of alcohol is also cured by it. Constipation—hence formation of gas, fermentation of undigested food, prolapse of rectum, stool passes unknowingly while passing urine are checked by it. It is of use in appendicitis, peritonitis, typhoid and other cases where chance of septic or infection has to be checked.

Potency: 30–200.

MYRISTICA SEBIFERA

Symptoms: This drug—being both a anti-septic and germicide—is chiefly used in treatment of bacterial problems such as abscess, ulcers and in all cases where pus has formed, so applicable in liver abscess, ulcers, appendicitis inflamed piles, fistula etc.

Potency: 3x–6.

NATRUM SULPHURICUM

Symptoms: This drug is applied to all sorts of liver and gall-bladder problems. Bileous vomit, bileous taste in mouth, bileous stool and diarrhea, stool passes while passing urine, heat and burning in stomach, large size of stool, dyspepsia, gas and mucus colitis are cured by it.

Potency: 6–30.

OLEANDER

Symptoms: This drug is useful in cases of indigestion, stool test shows undigested foods, rumbling of flatus in the lower abdomen, with burning sensation; also applied in hot water vomiting.

Potency: 6–30.

ORNITHOGALUM UMB

Symptoms: This drug is noted for its efficiency in treatment of gastric problems such as heaviness and pain around liver, hyperacidity, burning sensation, ulcer and cancer of the stomach, intestine leading to coffee coloured vomiting and presence of gas in the alimentary canal.

Potency: 1x–3x.

PTELEA

Symptoms: This drug is useful in lack of digestive powder leading to eructation, nausea, vomiting, feeling of heaviness in stomach, acidity, liver sore and pain and burning sensation in stomach, retraction of abdomen following pain.

Potency: 3x–30.

QUASSIA

Symptoms: Quassia is said to calm stomach inflammations and promote digestion by checking the action of acidity and gas. Gastric pain is relieved by its use. Dyspepsia, heart burn, frequent stool and preliminary stage of cirrhosis of liver.

Potency: 3x–3.

RAPHANUS

Symptoms: This drug is useful in problems associated with indigestion and constipation leading to accumulation of gas or loose stool and swelling of the abdomen. Also prescribed in eructation, vomiting, burning sensation in abdomen as a result of gas.

Potency: 6x–30.

ROBINA

Symptoms: Robina is prescribed in cases of hyperacidity, indigestion, flatulence. Bileous vomiting, stool and sour body smell are cases calling for its use.

Potency: 3x–6.

SCUTELLARIA LATERI

Symptoms: This drug is useful in spasms and pain originating with indigestion. Nausea, eructation, gas and gastric pain, bloating of abdomen, loose stool etc. call for its use.

Potency: 3x–6.

STRONTIA

Symptoms: Strontia is said to be effective in vomiting of pregnancy, dyspepsia, flatulence, acidity, continues urging to stool, rumbling in lower abdomen.

Potency: 6x–30.

TROMBIDUM

Symptoms: This drug is generally recommended in dysentery with much griping and burning sensation in stomach.

Potency: 6–30.

Some Symptoms and Medicines (Homeopathic)

1. To relieve diarrhea and prolapse of rectum—*Acacia Arabica* 3x.

2. To reduce swelling of spleen and piles—*Tamarix Dioica* 3x.

3. For bleeding piles—*Nyctanthes Arbour* 3x.

4. A good blood purifier, anti-septic for mouth wash. Killer of intestinal parasites also a purgative—*Solanum Xantho* 1x.

5. Retraction of lower intestine—*Indium Met* 30.

6. For fungal and bacterial infection—*Acetic acid, Acid Carb* 200.

7. Antacid in case of hyperacidity—*Robina, Bismuth* 6x.

8. Urge for speedy stool, rumbling in lower abdomen—*Castanea Vas* Q.

9. Once vomiting starts, even water is vomited out—*Gaultheria* Q.

10. Stomach swells up, patient bends forward with pain—*Curare* 30.

11. Rectum coming out—*Ferrum Phos* 12x.

12. Bad effect of drinking wine—*Asaram Euro* 3x.

13. Enlarged liver—*Yucca Filamentosa* 6x.

14. Dropsy due to enlarged liver and spleen—*Liatris Spi* 6.

15. Intestinal bleeding during typhoid—*Hydrastin Sulph* 3x.

16. To tone up rectum muscles—*Cal Phos* 12x, *Oxytroopis* 6x.

17. Gas and headache due to gas in bowels—*Onosmodium* 6.

18. Urge for stool after food—*Aurum Mur Nat* 6.

19. White colour of stool—*Aurum Mur Nat* or *Podophyllum* 6.

20. Stool not coming out despite great straining—*Polygonum* 3x.

21. Patient turns front and back with pain—*Piper Methy* 1x.

22. Fissure and Piles—*Paeonia Offi* 3x.

23. Stomach pain radiates backward—*Cochlearia* 3x.

24. Sticky Stool—-*Anthemis Nobelis* 3, *Platina* 6x.

25. Stool with Mucus—*Mag Mur* 6, *Hydrastis* 6x.

26. Difficulty in Swallowing—Merc-Bin-Iod, Argent Mel-30.

27. Stomatitis—*Cal Ars* 30, *Phytolecca* 1x (Gurgle), *Acid Mur* 200.

28. Sore Throat—*Hydrastis, Arsenic-Iod, Echinesia* 6.

29. Bowel obstruction, stool comes out from mouth—*Plumbum* 6 or refer to hospital.

30. Stomach pain, diarrhea of children during dentition—*Chamomilla* 6.

31. Bleeding Ulcer in Stomach—*Hydras Mur* 3x, *Geranium Mac* 1x.

32. Blood congestion in liver—*Euonymous* 3x.

33. White tongue—*Bryonia, Natrum Ars, Podophyllum* 30.

34. Lying senseless after diarrhea or pain—*Chloral Hydrate* 30, *Kali-Hydro* 6, *Nux-mus* 6.

35. To increase pulse—*Arsenic, Acid Hydro* 30.

36. Pain radiates to different parts—*Dioscorea, Mag Phos.*

37. Cholera in pregnancy—*Baptisa* 1x.

38. Stool comes and goes back—*Thuja, Hepar Sulph* 30.

39. Pain in stomach like electric shocks—*Thallium* 30.

40. Feeling of a lump in throat or stomach—*Argent Nit* 30, *Graphites* 200.

41. Constriction of anus, stool not coming out—*Plumbum* 30, *Ratanha* 6, *Graphites* 30.

42. Diarrhea with blood and mucus—*Merc-Dulchis* 6.

43. Stool as marble—*Mag Mur* 30, *China* 30, *Graphites* 30.

44. Burning hot gas from stomach to throat—*Lactic acid* 30.

45. Paralysis of Rectum—*Nux-vom* 30, *Thallium 30.*

46. Deficient Secretion of Gastric Juice—*Alnus, Berberis, Nux-vom.*

47. Digestion slow, feeling of heaviness after food—*Bismuth, Carboveg* 6x.

48. Hungry after food—*Cina, Chelidonium, Cal Carb, Lycopod* 30.

49. Increased appetite yet becoming bony—*Nat Mur, Iodium, Cal Phos* 6.

50. Pain immediately after eating—*Abies Nig, Belladona, Puls* 30.

51. Nausea from beer and water—*Arsenic, Kali Hydro* 30, *Kali Bich* 30.

52. Feeling as if stomach is pulled backward—*Plumbum Met* 30.

53. Feeling as if stomach is full of water—*Graphites, Abrotanum* 30.

54. Feeling of emptiness in stomach—*Hydrastis* 6.

55. Hands yellow nails flue—*Carboveg, Silicia, Nat Nit* 30.

56. Sour stool—*Rheum, Iris-vers* 6.

57. No desire for stool—*Hydrastis, Opium, Polygonum* 6.

58. Dilatation of stomach—*Hydras Mur* 6.